1

Optimal Strategies for Managing Hypertension: A Comprehensive Treatment Approach

Nathaniel R. Brogan

Table Of Contents

Chapter 1

I. Introduction to Hypertension

A. What is hypertension?

Hypertension, also known as high blood pressure, is a common medical condition characterized by elevated blood pressure levels in the arteries. It is a significant global health issue, affecting a large number of individuals worldwide.

Blood pressure is the force exerted by the blood against the walls of the arteries as the heart pumps it throughout the body. It is measured in millimeters of mercury (mmHg) and expressed as two numbers: systolic pressure over diastolic pressure. The systolic pressure represents the force when the heart contracts and pumps blood, while the diastolic pressure represents the force when the heart is at rest between beats.

Hypertension is typically diagnosed when a person consistently has a systolic pressure of 130 mmHg or higher and/or a diastolic pressure of 80 mmHg or higher. However, it is important to note that the diagnostic criteria and treatment targets may vary depending on guidelines and individual circumstances.

There are two main types of hypertension: primary (essential) hypertension and secondary hypertension.

Primary Hypertension: This is the most common form of hypertension, accounting for about 90-95% of cases. Primary hypertension tends to develop gradually over time and has no specific identifiable cause. It is influenced by a combination of genetic and environmental factors, such as age, family history, obesity, sedentary lifestyle, high salt intake, excessive alcohol consumption, and stress.

Secondary Hypertension: Secondary hypertension is caused by an underlying medical condition or external factors that contribute to high blood pressure. These conditions may include kidney disease, hormonal disorders (e.g., thyroid problems, adrenal gland disorders), certain medications (e.g., oral contraceptives, nonsteroidal anti-inflammatory drugs), sleep apnea, certain tumors, and drug abuse.

Hypertension is considered a significant risk factor for various health complications, including:

Cardiovascular Diseases: Prolonged high blood pressure can damage the arteries, leading to atherosclerosis (hardening and narrowing of the arteries), coronary artery disease, heart attack, heart failure, and arrhythmias.

Stroke: Hypertension increases the risk of stroke by damaging blood vessels in the brain or promoting the formation of blood clots that can block blood flow.

Kidney Disease: High blood pressure can damage the kidneys and impair their ability to filter waste and excess fluids from the body, potentially leading to chronic kidney disease or kidney failure.

Eye Problems: Hypertension can damage blood vessels in the eyes, causing vision problems or even blindness.

Other Complications: Hypertension can contribute to the development or worsening of other conditions, including peripheral artery disease, dementia, sexual dysfunction, and metabolic syndrome.

Managing hypertension involves a combination of lifestyle modifications and, if necessary, medications. Lifestyle changes include adopting a healthy diet (such as the DASH diet), reducing sodium intake, maintaining a healthy weight, engaging in regular physical activity, limiting alcohol consumption, and managing stress. Medications may be prescribed to lower blood pressure when lifestyle changes alone are insufficient.

Regular monitoring of blood pressure and routine medical check-ups are crucial for early detection, management, and prevention of complications associated with hypertension. It is essential for individuals with hypertension to work closely with healthcare professionals to develop a personalized treatment plan and maintain good overall cardiovascular health.

B. Prevalence and significance of hypertension

Hypertension, also known as high blood pressure, is a common medical condition that affects a significant portion of the global population. While I don't have access to real-time data, I can provide you with an overview of the prevalence of hypertension based on the information available up until September 2021. Please note that these figures may have changed since then. Here are some key points regarding the prevalence of hypertension:

1. Global Prevalence: Hypertension is a worldwide health concern. According to the World Health Organization (WHO), it is estimated that approximately 1.13 billion people worldwide have hypertension.

2. Age-related Prevalence: Hypertension becomes more prevalent as individuals age. The risk of developing hypertension increases with age due to various factors, such as reduced elasticity of blood vessels and overall cardiovascular health. However, hypertension can affect people of all age groups.

3. Regional Variations: The prevalence of hypertension varies across different regions. It is generally more prevalent in low- and middle-income countries compared to high-income

countries. This is partly due to differences in lifestyle, dietary habits, and access to healthcare.

4. Awareness and Control: Hypertension is often referred to as the "silent killer" because it may not cause noticeable symptoms initially. Therefore, many individuals with hypertension may remain unaware of their condition. Additionally, even when diagnosed, not all patients have their blood pressure adequately controlled. Proper management and lifestyle modifications are crucial to prevent complications.

5. Risk Factors: Several factors contribute to the development of hypertension, including genetics, sedentary lifestyle, poor dietary habits (high salt intake, low potassium intake), obesity, tobacco and alcohol use, stress, and certain chronic conditions like diabetes and kidney disease.

6. Complications: Hypertension, if left uncontrolled, can lead to serious health complications. It increases the risk of heart disease, stroke, kidney disease, and other cardiovascular conditions. Managing hypertension is essential to prevent these complications.

Remember that these figures are based on the information available up to September 2021, and the actual prevalence of hypertension may have changed. It's always advisable to refer to the most recent data from reputable health organizations and consult with healthcare professionals for accurate and up-to-date information.

Hypertension, or high blood pressure, is a significant medical condition with several important implications. Here are some key points highlighting the significance of hypertension:

1. Prevalence and Impact: Hypertension is highly prevalent worldwide and is a leading cause of cardiovascular diseases, including heart attacks, strokes, heart failure, and kidney disease. It is estimated to contribute to over 13% of global deaths.

2. Silent Nature: Hypertension is often referred to as the "silent killer" because it may not cause noticeable symptoms initially. Many individuals with hypertension remain unaware of their condition until it has already caused damage to their organs or led to a cardiovascular event. Regular blood pressure monitoring is crucial for early detection and management.

3. Major Risk Factor: Hypertension is a major risk factor for cardiovascular diseases. Persistently high blood pressure puts strain on the arteries and the heart, leading to increased risks of heart attacks, strokes, and other cardiovascular complications.

4. Impact on Organs: Uncontrolled hypertension can damage various organs in the body. The elevated pressure in the blood vessels can lead to the thickening and narrowing of arteries, reducing blood flow to vital organs like the heart, brain, and kidneys. This can result in heart disease, stroke, kidney disease, and other complications.

5. Economic Burden: Hypertension poses a significant economic burden on individuals, families, and healthcare systems. The costs associated with diagnosis, treatment, and management of hypertension, as well as the expenses related to its complications, place a substantial financial strain on healthcare systems and individuals alike.

6. Prevention and Management: Hypertension is largely preventable and manageable. Lifestyle modifications, including maintaining a healthy weight, regular physical activity, adopting a balanced diet (low in sodium and high in fruits and vegetables), limiting alcohol consumption, and avoiding tobacco use, can help prevent and manage hypertension. Medications may also be prescribed to control blood pressure when necessary.

7. Public Health Importance: Given the high prevalence and impact of hypertension, it is a significant public health concern. Public health initiatives and awareness campaigns play a crucial role in educating individuals about the

importance of blood pressure control, early detection, and adopting healthy lifestyle habits.

Managing hypertension is crucial for preventing its complications and improving overall health outcomes. Regular blood pressure monitoring, adherence to treatment plans, and lifestyle modifications are essential components of hypertension management. It is important to consult with healthcare professionals for personalized advice and treatment.

Chapter 2

II. Lifestyle Modifications

A. Dietary changes

Dietary changes can play a significant role in managing hypertension. Here are some key recommendations for modifying your diet to help control high blood pressure:

1. Reduce Sodium Intake: High sodium intake is strongly associated with hypertension. Limiting your sodium consumption can help lower blood pressure. Aim to consume less than 2,300 milligrams (mg) of sodium per day, and even lower if you have certain conditions like kidney disease. Avoid or minimize processed foods, canned soups, fast food, and salty snacks. Read food labels to identify hidden sources of sodium.

2. Increase Potassium-Rich Foods: Potassium helps counteract the effects of sodium and promote healthy blood pressure levels. Increase your intake of potassium-rich foods, such as fruits (bananas, oranges, melons), vegetables (leafy greens, potatoes, sweet potatoes), legumes (beans, lentils), and dairy products (low-fat milk, yogurt). Consult with your healthcare

provider if you have kidney problems or are on certain medications that require potassium restriction.

3. Adopt the DASH Diet: The Dietary Approaches to Stop Hypertension (DASH) diet has been shown to effectively lower blood pressure. It emphasizes fruits, vegetables, whole grains, lean proteins (such as poultry, fish, and beans), and low-fat dairy products. It also encourages reducing sodium, sugar, and saturated and trans fats. The DASH diet provides a well-balanced approach to nutrition and is rich in nutrients that support heart health.

4. Limit Saturated and Trans Fats: High intake of saturated and trans fats is associated with an increased risk of cardiovascular diseases. Choose lean sources of protein, such as skinless poultry, fish, legumes, and tofu. Replace saturated fats (found in fatty meats, full-fat dairy products, and tropical oils) with healthier fats like monounsaturated fats (found in olive oil, avocados, and nuts) and polyunsaturated fats (found in fatty fish, walnuts, and flaxseeds).

5. Increase Fiber Intake: Dietary fiber offers numerous health benefits, including helping to manage blood pressure. Increase your consumption of whole grains, fruits, vegetables, legumes, and nuts, as they are excellent sources of fiber. Aim for at least 25 to 30 grams of fiber per day.

6. Moderate Alcohol Consumption: Excessive alcohol intake can raise blood pressure and contribute to other health problems. If you choose to drink alcohol, do so in moderation. Moderate drinking is defined as up to one drink per day for women and up to two drinks per day for men.

7. Limit Added Sugars: Consuming excessive amounts of added sugars can lead to weight gain and increased blood pressure. Minimize your intake of sugary beverages, sweets, processed snacks, and desserts. Opt for healthier alternatives like fresh fruits when craving something sweet.

Remember that dietary changes alone may not be sufficient to control hypertension. It is important to combine them with regular physical activity, weight management, stress reduction, and any medications prescribed by your healthcare provider. Additionally, consult with a registered dietitian or healthcare professional to tailor dietary recommendations to your specific needs and health conditions.

1. Sodium restriction

Sodium restriction is a crucial dietary modification for managing hypertension. Excessive sodium intake can contribute to high blood pressure by causing fluid retention and increasing the volume of blood in the bloodstream. Here are some key recommendations for sodium restriction in the context of hypertension:

1. Daily Sodium Limit: The American Heart Association (AHA) and other health organizations generally recommend limiting sodium intake to less than 2,300 milligrams (mg) per day. However, for certain populations, such as individuals with hypertension, African Americans, and those with kidney disease, the recommended limit is often lower, typically around 1,500 mg per day.

2. Read Food Labels: Pay attention to food labels and select products that are low in sodium. Opt for items labeled as "low-sodium," "reduced sodium," or "no added salt." Compare different brands and choose those with lower sodium content.

3. Cook from Scratch: Preparing meals at home allows you to have better control over the sodium content of your food. Use fresh ingredients, herbs, and spices to enhance flavor instead

of relying on salt. Experiment with various seasonings and herbs to add taste to your dishes.

4. Minimize Processed Foods: Processed and packaged foods are often high in sodium. These include canned soups, frozen meals, deli meats, sauces, salad dressings, and snacks like chips and pretzels. Limit your consumption of these foods or choose low-sodium alternatives.

5. Be Aware of Hidden Sodium: Some foods may not taste salty but can still contain substantial amounts of sodium. Examples include bread, cheese, condiments (such as ketchup and soy sauce), pickles, and some breakfast cereals. Read labels carefully and choose low-sodium options when available.

6. Restaurant Choices: When dining out, it can be challenging to control sodium intake. Look for menu options that are labeled as low-sodium or ask for sauces and dressings on the side, so you can control the amount added to your meal. Requesting that your meal be prepared without added salt can also help reduce sodium content.

7. Rinse and Drain Canned Foods: If you use canned foods like beans or vegetables, rinsing them under water before consuming can help reduce their sodium content. Draining

and rinsing can remove a significant portion of the sodium in canned foods.

Remember, sodium restriction should be implemented in conjunction with an overall healthy diet and lifestyle modifications. It is important to work with your healthcare provider or a registered dietitian who can provide personalized guidance and help you manage your sodium intake based on your specific health needs and conditions.

2. DASH (Dietary Approaches to Stop Hypertension) diet

The Dietary Approaches to Stop Hypertension (DASH) diet is a dietary pattern specifically designed to lower blood pressure and promote heart health. It emphasizes a balanced and nutrient-rich approach to eating. Here are the key features and recommendations of the DASH diet:

1. Fruits and Vegetables: The DASH diet encourages the consumption of a variety of fruits and vegetables. Aim for 4 to 5 servings of fruits and vegetables each day. Include fresh, frozen, or canned options without added sugars or salt. These foods provide essential vitamins, minerals, fiber, and antioxidants.

2. Whole Grains: Choose whole grains instead of refined grains. Include foods like whole wheat, brown rice, oats, quinoa, and whole grain bread and pasta. Whole grains are higher in fiber and nutrients compared to refined grains.

3. Lean Protein: Opt for lean protein sources such as skinless poultry, fish, beans, lentils, and tofu. These foods are lower in saturated fat compared to fatty meats. Aim for 2 to 3 servings of protein per day.

4. Low-Fat Dairy: Include low-fat or fat-free dairy products like milk, yogurt, and cheese in your diet. They provide calcium, potassium, and protein. Aim for 2 to 3 servings of dairy per day. If you have lactose intolerance or avoid dairy, consider alternative sources of calcium and fortified non-dairy milk.

5. Nuts, Seeds, and Legumes: These are good sources of plant-based protein, healthy fats, and fiber. Include options like almonds, walnuts, chia seeds, flaxseeds, and various legumes (beans, lentils, chickpeas) in your diet. However, be mindful of portion sizes due to their calorie content.

6. Limited Sodium Intake: The DASH diet recommends reducing sodium intake to help lower blood pressure. Aim for no more than 2,300 milligrams (mg) of sodium per day. However, for individuals with hypertension or at higher risk, the recommended limit is often around 1,500 mg per day. Choose low-sodium or no-added-salt options, minimize processed foods, and limit the use of table salt.

7. Limit Saturated and Trans Fats: The DASH diet encourages reducing saturated fats and eliminating trans fats. Limit the consumption of fatty meats, full-fat dairy products, fried foods, and foods containing partially hydrogenated oils. Instead, opt for healthier fats like monounsaturated fats (olive

oil, avocados) and polyunsaturated fats (fatty fish, nuts, seeds).

8. Moderate Sugar Intake: The DASH diet suggests limiting added sugars and sugary beverages. Reduce your consumption of sugary snacks, desserts, sodas, and fruit juices. Instead, satisfy your sweet tooth with fresh fruits.

9. Portion Control and Caloric Balance: Although the DASH diet does not explicitly focus on calorie counting, portion control and maintaining a healthy weight are important aspects. Be mindful of portion sizes and balance your caloric intake with physical activity to achieve or maintain a healthy weight.

Remember, the DASH diet is not a quick fix but a long-term approach to healthy eating. It is advisable to consult with a registered dietitian or healthcare professional to tailor the DASH diet to your specific needs, health conditions, and dietary preferences. They can provide personalized guidance and support in implementing the diet successfully.

3. Potassium-rich foods

Including potassium-rich foods in your diet can be beneficial for managing hypertension. Potassium helps counteract the effects of sodium, relaxes blood vessels, and supports healthy blood pressure levels. Here are some examples of potassium-rich foods that you can incorporate into your diet:

1. Fruits: Many fruits are excellent sources of potassium. Some potassium-rich fruits include bananas, oranges, kiwis, avocados, cantaloupes, apricots, and strawberries.

2. Vegetables: Numerous vegetables are high in potassium. Consider adding spinach, kale, Swiss chard, broccoli, Brussels sprouts, sweet potatoes, potatoes, tomatoes, and mushrooms to your meals.

3. Legumes: Legumes such as beans, lentils, and peas are not only rich in potassium but also provide fiber and protein. Incorporate kidney beans, black beans, chickpeas, lentils, and edamame into your diet.

4. Nuts and Seeds: Nuts and seeds are good sources of potassium, healthy fats, and other beneficial nutrients. Include almonds, pistachios, walnuts, flaxseeds, and chia seeds in your snacks or meals.

5. Dairy Products: Dairy products like milk, yogurt, and cheese are potassium-rich. Opt for low-fat or fat-free varieties to minimize saturated fat intake.

6. Fish: Some fish varieties are high in potassium and heart-healthy omega-3 fatty acids. Consider including salmon, mackerel, tuna, and sardines in your diet.

7. Meats: Lean meats, such as chicken and turkey breast, are sources of potassium. However, they generally contain lower amounts of potassium compared to plant-based sources.

8. Other Sources: Additional potassium-rich options include soy products (tofu, tempeh), whole grains (brown rice, quinoa), and certain beverages like coconut water and orange juice.

Remember that individual potassium needs may vary based on factors such as age, sex, and underlying health conditions. It is advisable to consult with your healthcare provider or a registered dietitian to determine the appropriate potassium intake for your specific situation. They can provide personalized recommendations and help you incorporate potassium-rich foods into a well-balanced diet.

4. Reduced alcohol consumption

Reducing alcohol consumption is an important lifestyle modification for managing hypertension. Excessive alcohol intake can raise blood pressure and increase the risk of cardiovascular complications. Here are some key points to consider regarding alcohol consumption and hypertension:

1. Moderate Drinking Guidelines: Moderate alcohol consumption is generally defined as up to one drink per day for women and up to two drinks per day for men. This refers to the standard drink size, which typically contains about 14 grams of pure alcohol. It's important to note that these guidelines are not meant to encourage non-drinkers to start drinking for health benefits.

2. Blood Pressure Effects: Drinking excessive amounts of alcohol can lead to a temporary increase in blood pressure. Over time, chronic heavy drinking can contribute to the development of hypertension. It's recommended to limit alcohol intake to help manage blood pressure levels.

3. Individual Sensitivity: People's reactions to alcohol can vary. Some individuals may experience a greater blood pressure response to alcohol compared to others. Factors like

age, genetics, overall health, and the presence of other risk factors for hypertension should be taken into account.

4. Alcohol and Medications: If you are taking medications to manage hypertension or other health conditions, it's essential to consult your healthcare provider about the potential interactions between alcohol and your medications. Alcohol can interfere with the effectiveness and safety of certain medications.

5. Other Health Risks: Excessive alcohol consumption not only increases the risk of hypertension but also contributes to various other health problems, including liver disease, heart disease, stroke, certain types of cancer, and addiction. Limiting alcohol intake can help reduce the risk of these health complications.

6. Strategies for Reducing Alcohol Intake: If you find it challenging to reduce your alcohol consumption, consider the following strategies:

  - Set realistic goals: Start by gradually reducing your alcohol intake rather than quitting abruptly.
  - Seek support: Reach out to supportive friends, family members, or support groups if you need help in reducing or quitting alcohol.

- Find alternatives: Engage in activities or hobbies that do not revolve around alcohol. Find healthier ways to relax and unwind.

- Avoid triggers: Identify situations or environments that encourage excessive drinking and try to avoid them.

- Seek professional help: If you're struggling to reduce your alcohol intake or if you have an alcohol dependency, consider seeking guidance from healthcare professionals or addiction specialists.

It's important to remember that individual circumstances may vary, and it's always advisable to consult with your healthcare provider for personalized advice and guidance on alcohol consumption, especially if you have hypertension or other health concerns.

B. Weight management

Weight management plays a crucial role in managing hypertension, as excess weight and obesity are significant risk factors for developing high blood pressure. Losing weight and maintaining a healthy weight can help reduce blood pressure levels and improve overall cardiovascular health. Here are some key points to consider regarding weight management for hypertension:

1. Body Mass Index (BMI): Start by determining your BMI, which is a measure of body fat based on height and weight. A BMI between 18.5 and 24.9 is considered within the normal weight range. If your BMI is higher, it indicates that you may be overweight or obese, increasing your risk of hypertension.

2. Set Realistic Goals: Aim for gradual and sustainable weight loss rather than quick and drastic measures. Losing even a modest amount of weight can have significant benefits for blood pressure and overall health.

3. Caloric Balance: Weight management involves achieving a caloric balance by consuming an appropriate number of calories to support your daily activities and energy needs. This typically involves consuming fewer calories than you burn. It's important to consult with a healthcare professional or

registered dietitian to determine a suitable calorie intake based on your specific needs and goals.

4. Healthy Eating Habits: Adopting a well-balanced and nutritious diet is essential for weight management. Include plenty of fruits, vegetables, whole grains, lean proteins, and healthy fats in your meals. Avoid or limit high-calorie and processed foods that are often low in nutritional value.

5. Portion Control: Be mindful of portion sizes to avoid overeating. Use smaller plates and bowls to help control portion sizes and prevent excessive calorie intake. Listen to your body's hunger and fullness cues.

6. Regular Physical Activity: Engage in regular physical activity to support weight loss and overall cardiovascular health. Aim for at least 150 minutes of moderate-intensity aerobic exercise or 75 minutes of vigorous-intensity aerobic exercise per week, along with strength training exercises at least twice a week. Consult with your healthcare provider before starting a new exercise program.

7. Behavior and Lifestyle Changes: Adopt healthy behaviors and lifestyle habits that support weight management. This includes getting adequate sleep, managing stress, limiting alcohol consumption, and avoiding smoking.

8. Support and Accountability: Seek support from family, friends, or support groups to help you stay motivated and accountable on your weight management journey. Consider working with a registered dietitian or a healthcare professional who can provide personalized guidance and support.

It's important to note that weight management is a long-term commitment, and results may vary from person to person. The focus should be on overall health improvement rather than solely on the number on the scale. Consulting with a healthcare professional can provide personalized guidance tailored to your specific needs, health conditions, and preferences.

1. Importance of weight loss

Weight loss is of great importance for hypertensive patients because it can significantly improve their blood pressure control and overall cardiovascular health. Here are the key reasons why weight loss is crucial for individuals with hypertension:

1. Blood Pressure Reduction: Excess weight and obesity are strongly associated with an increased risk of developing hypertension. Losing weight can lead to a decrease in blood pressure levels, both systolic and diastolic. Studies have shown that even modest weight loss can have a significant impact on blood pressure reduction.

2. Reduced Medication Dependency: Weight loss can potentially reduce or even eliminate the need for antihypertensive medications in some cases. By achieving and maintaining a healthy weight, individuals may be able to manage their blood pressure through lifestyle modifications alone, or with lower doses of medication, leading to fewer side effects and healthcare costs.

3. Lower Risk of Cardiovascular Complications: Hypertension is a major risk factor for various cardiovascular diseases, including heart disease, stroke, and heart failure. Weight loss helps lower this risk by improving blood pressure

control, reducing strain on the heart and blood vessels, and improving overall cardiovascular function.

4. Improved Insulin Sensitivity: Obesity and hypertension are often linked with insulin resistance and an increased risk of developing type 2 diabetes. Weight loss can enhance insulin sensitivity, leading to better blood sugar control and a decreased risk of developing diabetes or better management of existing diabetes.

5. Health Benefits Beyond Blood Pressure: Weight loss has numerous additional health benefits. It can improve lipid profiles by lowering total cholesterol, LDL cholesterol (often referred to as "bad" cholesterol), and triglyceride levels while increasing HDL cholesterol (often referred to as "good" cholesterol). Weight loss also contributes to better overall cardiovascular fitness, improved lung function, reduced joint stress, and enhanced psychological well-being.

6. Synergistic Effects with Other Lifestyle Modifications: Weight loss complements other lifestyle modifications recommended for managing hypertension, such as adopting a healthy diet (e.g., DASH diet), engaging in regular physical activity, limiting alcohol consumption, and reducing sodium intake. Combining weight loss with these lifestyle changes can have a synergistic effect on blood pressure control and overall health improvement.

It's important to note that weight loss should be approached in a safe and sustainable manner. Gradual weight loss, aiming for a loss of about 1-2 pounds per week, is generally recommended. Consulting with a healthcare professional or registered dietitian is advisable to develop an individualized weight loss plan tailored to your specific needs, health conditions, and preferences.

Weight loss is a long-term commitment, and maintaining a healthy weight requires ongoing lifestyle changes. However, the benefits of weight loss for individuals with hypertension are significant and can contribute to improved blood pressure control, reduced risk of cardiovascular complications, and better overall health outcomes.

2.   Physical activity recommendations

Physical activity is an important component of managing hypertension and promoting overall cardiovascular health. Regular exercise can help lower blood pressure, improve heart health, enhance blood flow, and contribute to weight management. Here are some recommendations for physical activity for individuals with hypertension:

1. Consult with Your Healthcare Provider: Before starting any exercise program, it's important to consult with your healthcare provider, especially if you have underlying health conditions or are currently taking medications. They can provide personalized guidance and recommendations based on your specific situation.

2. Aim for Aerobic Exercise: Engage in aerobic exercises that raise your heart rate and increase your breathing. Examples of aerobic exercises include brisk walking, jogging, cycling, swimming, dancing, aerobics classes, and using cardio machines like treadmills or ellipticals. Aim for at least 150 minutes of moderate-intensity aerobic exercise or 75 minutes of vigorous-intensity aerobic exercise per week. You can divide the time into shorter sessions throughout the week if needed.

3. Start Slow and Gradually Increase Intensity: If you are new to exercise or have been inactive for a while, it's important to start slowly and gradually increase the intensity and duration of your workouts. Begin with shorter durations and lower intensities, and as you become more comfortable and fit, gradually increase the intensity and duration of your exercises.

4. Incorporate Strength Training: Include strength training exercises at least two days per week. Strength training helps build muscle strength, which can support overall cardiovascular health. Use resistance bands, free weights, weight machines, or perform bodyweight exercises like squats, lunges, push-ups, and planks. Focus on targeting major muscle groups, and allow for rest days between sessions to allow for muscle recovery.

5. Monitor Intensity: Pay attention to your perceived exertion level during exercise. Aim for a moderate intensity level where you feel somewhat breathless but still able to carry on a conversation. Avoid overexertion and pushing yourself too hard, especially if you have not been physically active.

6. Listen to Your Body: Be mindful of any signs or symptoms that may indicate you need to modify or stop your exercise session. If you experience chest pain, severe shortness of

breath, dizziness, lightheadedness, or any other concerning symptoms, stop exercising and seek medical attention.

7. Stay Consistent: Consistency is key when it comes to physical activity. Aim for regular exercise sessions throughout the week rather than sporadic intense workouts. Find activities you enjoy and make them a part of your routine to increase the likelihood of long-term adherence.

8. Stay Hydrated: Drink plenty of water before, during, and after exercise to stay hydrated, especially in hot and humid environments.

Remember, individual fitness levels and preferences may vary, so it's important to find activities that you enjoy and are suitable for your specific needs. Working with a certified fitness professional or physical therapist can provide additional guidance and support in developing a safe and effective exercise program tailored to your needs and goals.

C. Smoking cessation

Smoking cessation is crucial for hypertensive patients as smoking is a major risk factor for the development and progression of hypertension, as well as various cardiovascular diseases. Quitting smoking offers numerous benefits for blood pressure control and overall health. Here are the key reasons why smoking cessation is important for individuals with hypertension:

1. Blood Pressure Control: Smoking tobacco leads to an immediate and temporary increase in blood pressure, as well as long-term damage to blood vessels. By quitting smoking, blood pressure levels can be significantly lowered, reducing the risk of complications associated with hypertension.

2. Reduced Risk of Cardiovascular Diseases: Hypertension and smoking together greatly increase the risk of heart disease, stroke, and other cardiovascular conditions. By quitting smoking, individuals can lower their risk of these serious health complications.

3. Improved Medication Effectiveness: Smoking can affect the efficacy of certain medications used to manage hypertension. Quitting smoking can enhance the effectiveness

of antihypertensive medications, allowing for better blood pressure control.

4. Lung and Respiratory Health: Smoking damages the lungs and respiratory system, leading to conditions such as chronic obstructive pulmonary disease (COPD) and lung cancer. By quitting smoking, individuals can improve their lung function and reduce the risk of respiratory complications.

5. Reduced Inflammation and Oxidative Stress: Smoking increases inflammation and oxidative stress in the body, which can contribute to the development and progression of hypertension and other chronic diseases. Quitting smoking helps reduce these harmful effects, promoting overall health and well-being.

6. Lower Risk of Secondhand Smoke Exposure: Quitting smoking not only benefits the individual but also protects those around them from the harmful effects of secondhand smoke. Secondhand smoke exposure is also linked to an increased risk of hypertension and cardiovascular diseases.

7. Improved Exercise Capacity: Smoking impairs lung function and reduces exercise capacity. By quitting smoking, individuals can improve their lung health and respiratory function, allowing for better exercise tolerance and overall physical fitness.

Quitting smoking can be challenging, but numerous resources and strategies are available to support individuals in their journey to become smoke-free:

- Nicotine Replacement Therapy (NRT): NRT products, such as nicotine patches, gum, lozenges, inhalers, and nasal sprays, can help manage nicotine withdrawal symptoms and cravings.

- Medications: Certain medications, such as bupropion and varenicline, can be prescribed by healthcare professionals to aid in smoking cessation.

- Behavioral Support: Seek support from healthcare professionals, counselors, or support groups that specialize in smoking cessation. Behavioral interventions, such as counseling or cognitive-behavioral therapy, can greatly increase the chances of successful quitting.

- Lifestyle Changes: Adopting a healthier lifestyle can help manage cravings and reduce the temptation to smoke. Engaging in regular physical activity, practicing stress-reduction techniques (e.g., deep breathing, meditation), and maintaining a well-balanced diet can support smoking cessation efforts.

Remember, quitting smoking is a journey that may involve multiple attempts. It's important to stay motivated and persistent. Even reducing the number of cigarettes smoked or the duration of smoking can have health benefits. Seek support from healthcare professionals who can provide personalized guidance and resources to help you quit smoking successfully.

Chapter 3

III. Pharmacological Treatment

Pharmacological treatment is often recommended for hypertensive patients to help control blood pressure and reduce the risk of cardiovascular complications. The specific medications prescribed will depend on factors such as the severity of hypertension, presence of other medical conditions, and individual patient characteristics. Here are some commonly used classes of medications for treating hypertension:

1. Angiotensin-Converting Enzyme (ACE) Inhibitors: ACE inhibitors block the action of an enzyme that produces a substance called angiotensin II, which causes blood vessels to narrow and constrict. By inhibiting this enzyme, ACE inhibitors help relax blood vessels, lower blood pressure, and reduce the workload on the heart. Examples include lisinopril, enalapril, and ramipril.

2. Angiotensin II Receptor Blockers (ARBs): ARBs work by blocking the receptors for angiotensin II, preventing its action on blood vessels. Like ACE inhibitors, ARBs help dilate

blood vessels and lower blood pressure. They are often prescribed as an alternative to ACE inhibitors, especially for individuals who cannot tolerate ACE inhibitors due to side effects. Examples include losartan, valsartan, and irbesartan.

3. Diuretics: Diuretics, also known as water pills, help eliminate excess sodium and water from the body, reducing the volume of blood and lowering blood pressure. They are often used as first-line treatment for hypertension. There are different types of diuretics, including thiazide diuretics (e.g., hydrochlorothiazide), loop diuretics (e.g., furosemide), and potassium-sparing diuretics (e.g., spironolactone).

4. Calcium Channel Blockers (CCBs): CCBs block the entry of calcium into the smooth muscle cells of blood vessels, causing them to relax and widen. This results in lowered blood pressure. CCBs can also have a direct effect on the heart by reducing its workload and decreasing heart rate. Examples of CCBs include amlodipine, diltiazem, and verapamil.

5. Beta-Blockers: Beta-blockers work by blocking the effects of adrenaline (epinephrine) on the heart, causing the heart to beat more slowly and with less force. This reduces blood pressure and helps lower the heart's workload. Beta-blockers may also be prescribed for individuals with certain heart

conditions, such as coronary artery disease or heart failure. Examples include metoprolol, atenolol, and propranolol.

6. Other Medications: In some cases, other medications may be prescribed to manage hypertension, depending on individual needs and circumstances. These may include alpha-blockers, central alpha agonists, direct renin inhibitors, or vasodilators.

It's important to note that medication choices and combinations will vary based on individual patient characteristics. Healthcare professionals will carefully evaluate each patient's medical history, blood pressure readings, and any concurrent conditions to determine the most appropriate medication regimen.

Regular monitoring of blood pressure and close follow-up with healthcare providers are essential to ensure that medications are effectively controlling blood pressure and to make any necessary adjustments to the treatment plan. Compliance with prescribed medications and any lifestyle modifications recommended by healthcare professionals is crucial for the optimal management of hypertension.

A. First-line antihypertensive medications

First-line antihypertensive medications are typically prescribed as initial treatment options for hypertensive patients. These medications are commonly recommended due to their effectiveness, safety profile, and evidence-based guidelines. The choice of first-line medication may vary based on individual patient characteristics and any coexisting medical conditions. Here are some commonly prescribed first-line antihypertensive medication classes:

1. Thiazide Diuretics: Thiazide diuretics are often recommended as the first-line treatment for hypertension, particularly for patients without other compelling indications. They help reduce blood pressure by promoting diuresis (increased urine production) and decreasing the volume of fluid in the blood vessels. Examples include hydrochlorothiazide, chlorthalidone, and indapamide.

2. Angiotensin-Converting Enzyme (ACE) Inhibitors: ACE inhibitors are another commonly prescribed first-line option. They block the action of the enzyme that converts angiotensin I to angiotensin II, leading to blood vessel relaxation and decreased blood pressure. ACE inhibitors are especially beneficial for patients with diabetes, heart failure, or chronic

kidney disease. Examples include lisinopril, enalapril, and ramipril.

3. Angiotensin II Receptor Blockers (ARBs): ARBs are often prescribed as an alternative to ACE inhibitors, particularly for patients who cannot tolerate ACE inhibitors due to side effects. They block the receptors that angiotensin II binds to, resulting in blood vessel relaxation and lowered blood pressure. ARBs are also beneficial for patients with certain comorbidities such as heart failure, diabetes, or chronic kidney disease. Examples include losartan, valsartan, and candesartan.

4. Calcium Channel Blockers (CCBs): CCBs are effective at lowering blood pressure by blocking the entry of calcium into the smooth muscle cells of blood vessels, causing them to relax and dilate. CCBs can also have a direct effect on the heart, reducing its workload and heart rate. They are particularly useful for patients with coexisting conditions such as angina or certain arrhythmias. Examples include amlodipine, diltiazem, and verapamil.

It's important to note that individual patient factors, such as age, race, comorbidities, and medication tolerability, may influence the choice of first-line medication. Additionally, combination therapy or adjustments to the treatment plan may be necessary if blood pressure targets are not achieved with monotherapy.

The selection of first-line antihypertensive medication should be made in consultation with a healthcare professional who will consider the patient's specific medical history, blood pressure readings, and individual needs to determine the most appropriate treatment plan. Regular monitoring and follow-up visits are crucial to evaluate the effectiveness of the medication and make any necessary adjustments.

1. Diuretics

Diuretics are a class of medications commonly used in the treatment of hypertension. They help lower blood pressure by increasing the excretion of sodium and water from the body, resulting in reduced blood volume and decreased pressure on the blood vessel walls. Diuretics are often prescribed as first-line treatment for hypertension and can be used alone or in combination with other antihypertensive medications. Here are the different types of diuretics used for hypertensive patients:

1. Thiazide Diuretics: Thiazide diuretics are one of the most commonly prescribed types of diuretics for hypertension. They work by inhibiting the reabsorption of sodium and chloride in the kidneys, leading to increased urine production and reduced fluid volume. Thiazide diuretics are effective in lowering blood pressure and are often used as first-line therapy. Examples include hydrochlorothiazide, chlorthalidone, and indapamide.

2. Loop Diuretics: Loop diuretics are more potent than thiazide diuretics and are usually reserved for patients with more severe hypertension or those with reduced kidney function. They inhibit the reabsorption of sodium, chloride, and water in the loop of Henle, a part of the kidney tubules.

Loop diuretics are useful when there is resistance to other diuretics or when significant fluid retention is present. Examples include furosemide, bumetanide, and torsemide.

3. Potassium-Sparing Diuretics: Potassium-sparing diuretics are diuretics that help eliminate sodium while sparing the loss of potassium. They work by blocking the action of aldosterone, a hormone that promotes sodium retention and potassium excretion. Potassium-sparing diuretics are often used in combination with thiazide or loop diuretics to counteract the potassium loss associated with those medications. Examples include spironolactone, eplerenone, and amiloride.

Diuretics are generally well-tolerated and can effectively lower blood pressure. However, it's important to monitor certain factors when using diuretics for hypertension:

- Electrolyte Levels: Diuretics can affect electrolyte levels, particularly potassium and sodium. Regular monitoring of these electrolytes is necessary, especially when using thiazide or loop diuretics. Potassium-sparing diuretics help prevent excessive potassium loss.

- Blood Pressure and Fluid Balance: Monitoring blood pressure and assessing fluid balance is important to ensure optimal management of hypertension and prevent complications associated with excessive fluid loss.

- Kidney Function: Diuretics may affect kidney function, so monitoring kidney function through regular blood tests is essential, especially when using loop diuretics or in patients with pre-existing kidney disease.

It's important to follow the prescribed dosage and any additional recommendations provided by your healthcare professional when taking diuretics. They will determine the most appropriate type and dose of diuretic based on your individual needs, medical history, and response to treatment. Regular follow-up visits with your healthcare provider are crucial to monitor the effectiveness of the medication and make any necessary adjustments.

2. Angiotensin-converting enzyme (ACE) inhibitors

Angiotensin-converting enzyme (ACE) inhibitors are a class of medications commonly prescribed for the treatment of hypertension. They work by blocking the activity of an enzyme called angiotensin-converting enzyme, which plays a role in the production of a hormone called angiotensin II. By inhibiting the production of angiotensin II, ACE inhibitors help relax and widen the blood vessels, leading to a decrease in blood pressure. Here are some key points about ACE inhibitors for hypertensive patients:

1. Mechanism of Action: ACE inhibitors block the conversion of angiotensin I to angiotensin II. Angiotensin II is a potent vasoconstrictor, meaning it narrows the blood vessels and increases blood pressure. By inhibiting its production, ACE inhibitors promote vasodilation, reduce peripheral resistance, and lower blood pressure.

2. Blood Pressure Control: ACE inhibitors are effective in lowering blood pressure and are commonly used as first-line treatment for hypertension. They are particularly beneficial for patients with certain conditions such as diabetes, heart failure, or chronic kidney disease, as they can help protect against kidney damage and reduce the risk of cardiovascular events.

3. Cardioprotective Effects: ACE inhibitors have additional benefits beyond blood pressure control. They are known to have cardioprotective effects and are often prescribed for patients with heart conditions such as heart failure or previous heart attacks. ACE inhibitors can help improve cardiac function, reduce strain on the heart, and prevent the remodeling of heart muscle.

4. Kidney Protection: ACE inhibitors help protect the kidneys by dilating the blood vessels in the kidneys and reducing the pressure within the kidney filters (glomeruli). They are often used to manage hypertension in patients with chronic kidney disease to slow down the progression of kidney damage.

5. Combination Therapy: ACE inhibitors are often prescribed in combination with other antihypertensive medications, such as diuretics or calcium channel blockers, to achieve better blood pressure control. Combination therapy may be necessary in patients with more severe hypertension or those who do not achieve adequate blood pressure reduction with a single medication.

6. Side Effects: While ACE inhibitors are generally well-tolerated, they can cause side effects in some individuals. Common side effects may include a dry cough, dizziness, headache, fatigue, or skin rash. Less commonly, ACE

inhibitors can cause a potentially serious side effect called angioedema, which involves swelling of the face, lips, tongue, or throat and requires immediate medical attention.

7. Precautions: ACE inhibitors should be used with caution in patients with a history of angioedema, kidney problems, or high levels of potassium in the blood. They are generally not recommended during pregnancy due to potential harm to the developing fetus.

It's important to take ACE inhibitors exactly as prescribed by your healthcare provider. Regular follow-up visits are essential to monitor blood pressure, kidney function, and any potential side effects. Your healthcare provider will determine the most appropriate medication, dose, and treatment plan based on your individual needs, medical history, and response to treatment.

3. Angiotensin II receptor blockers (ARBs)

Angiotensin II receptor blockers (ARBs) are a class of medications commonly prescribed for the treatment of hypertension. ARBs work by blocking the action of angiotensin II, a hormone that constricts blood vessels and increases blood pressure. By blocking the receptors to which angiotensin II binds, ARBs help relax and widen the blood vessels, resulting in a decrease in blood pressure. Here are some key points about ARBs for hypertensive patients:

1. Mechanism of Action: ARBs selectively block the angiotensin II receptors, specifically the type 1 (AT1) receptors. By doing so, they prevent angiotensin II from exerting its vasoconstrictive effects on the blood vessels, resulting in vasodilation and reduced blood pressure.

2. Blood Pressure Control: ARBs are effective in lowering blood pressure and are commonly used as first-line treatment for hypertension. They are particularly beneficial for patients with certain conditions such as diabetes, heart failure, or chronic kidney disease, as they can help protect against kidney damage and reduce the risk of cardiovascular events.

3. Similar to ACE Inhibitors: ARBs work on the same pathway as angiotensin-converting enzyme (ACE) inhibitors,

but they act at a different point. While ACE inhibitors block the production of angiotensin II, ARBs directly block its receptors. Both classes of medications have similar blood pressure-lowering effects, but ARBs are often prescribed as an alternative for patients who cannot tolerate ACE inhibitors due to side effects such as cough.

4. Cardioprotective Effects: Like ACE inhibitors, ARBs have additional benefits beyond blood pressure control. They have cardioprotective effects and are often prescribed for patients with heart conditions such as heart failure or previous heart attacks. ARBs can help improve cardiac function, reduce strain on the heart, and prevent the remodeling of heart muscle.

5. Kidney Protection: ARBs also have a protective effect on the kidneys. By dilating the blood vessels in the kidneys and reducing the pressure within the kidney filters (glomeruli), they help protect against kidney damage. ARBs are commonly used in patients with chronic kidney disease or proteinuria (excessive protein in the urine).

6. Combination Therapy: ARBs can be prescribed as monotherapy or in combination with other antihypertensive medications to achieve better blood pressure control. Combination therapy may be necessary in patients with more

severe hypertension or those who do not achieve adequate blood pressure reduction with a single medication.

7. Side Effects: ARBs are generally well-tolerated, and side effects are uncommon. Some individuals may experience dizziness, fatigue, or mild allergic reactions. They are usually less likely to cause a dry cough compared to ACE inhibitors. However, like ACE inhibitors, ARBs can rarely cause angioedema (swelling of the face, lips, tongue, or throat) and should be discontinued if this occurs.

8. Precautions: ARBs should be used with caution in patients with a history of angioedema, kidney problems, or high levels of potassium in the blood. They are generally not recommended during pregnancy due to potential harm to the developing fetus.

It's important to take ARBs exactly as prescribed by your healthcare provider. Regular follow-up visits are essential to monitor blood pressure, kidney function, and any potential side effects. Your healthcare provider will determine the most appropriate medication, dose, and treatment plan based on your individual needs, medical history, and response to treatment.

4. Calcium channel blockers (CCBs)

Calcium channel blockers (CCBs) are a class of medications commonly prescribed for the treatment of hypertension. CCBs work by blocking the entry of calcium into the smooth muscle cells of blood vessels, resulting in relaxation and dilation of the blood vessels. This leads to a decrease in peripheral resistance and a reduction in blood pressure. Here are some key points about CCBs for hypertensive patients:

1. Mechanism of Action: CCBs block calcium channels in the smooth muscle cells of blood vessels, preventing the entry of calcium ions. This inhibits the contraction of the muscle cells, leading to relaxation and dilation of the blood vessels. By reducing peripheral resistance, CCBs help lower blood pressure.

2. Blood Pressure Control: CCBs are effective in lowering blood pressure and are commonly used as first-line treatment for hypertension. They are particularly useful in patients with coexisting conditions such as angina (chest pain), certain arrhythmias, or migraine headaches.

3. Types of CCBs: There are two main types of CCBs: dihydropyridine and non-dihydropyridine.

- Dihydropyridine CCBs: This type of CCB primarily acts on the blood vessels, causing vasodilation and lowering blood pressure. Examples include amlodipine, nifedipine, and felodipine.

- Non-dihydropyridine CCBs: This type of CCB not only acts on the blood vessels but also affects the heart's electrical conduction system. They are often used in patients with certain heart conditions, such as atrial fibrillation or hypertrophic cardiomyopathy. Examples include verapamil and diltiazem.

4. Heart Rate and Cardiac Effects: Non-dihydropyridine CCBs, specifically verapamil and diltiazem, can lower heart rate and are beneficial for patients with conditions involving rapid heart rates or certain types of arrhythmias. Dihydropyridine CCBs have minimal effects on heart rate and are preferred for their vasodilatory properties.

5. Combination Therapy: CCBs can be used alone or in combination with other antihypertensive medications to achieve better blood pressure control. They are often combined with other classes of medications such as diuretics, ACE inhibitors, or ARBs.

6. Side Effects: CCBs are generally well-tolerated, but like any medication, they can cause side effects in some

individuals. Common side effects may include dizziness, headache, flushing, peripheral edema (swelling of the extremities), and constipation. Non-dihydropyridine CCBs can also cause bradycardia (low heart rate) and heart block.

7. Precautions: CCBs should be used with caution in patients with certain medical conditions, such as heart failure or impaired liver function. They may interact with other medications, so it's important to inform your healthcare provider about all the medications you are taking.

It's important to take CCBs exactly as prescribed by your healthcare provider. Regular follow-up visits are essential to monitor blood pressure, heart rate, and any potential side effects. Your healthcare provider will determine the most appropriate medication, dose, and treatment plan based on your individual needs, medical history, and response to treatment.

5. Beta blockers

Beta blockers are a class of medications commonly prescribed for the treatment of hypertension. They work by blocking the action of adrenaline and other stress hormones on beta receptors in the body. By doing so, beta blockers reduce the effects of these hormones, leading to a decrease in heart rate and the force of contraction, resulting in lower blood pressure. Here are some key points about beta blockers for hypertensive patients:

1. Mechanism of Action: Beta blockers block the beta receptors in the body, specifically beta-1 receptors primarily located in the heart. By blocking these receptors, beta blockers reduce the effects of adrenaline and other stress hormones on the heart, leading to decreased heart rate and contractility. This results in lowered blood pressure.

2. Blood Pressure Control: Beta blockers are effective in lowering blood pressure and are commonly used as first-line treatment for hypertension. They are particularly beneficial for patients with certain conditions such as prior heart attacks, heart failure, or certain arrhythmias.

3. Heart Rate and Cardiac Effects: Beta blockers reduce heart rate, making them useful in conditions where the heart rate

needs to be controlled, such as certain types of arrhythmias or when there is an excessive increase in heart rate during physical or emotional stress. By reducing the force of contraction, beta blockers also help reduce the workload on the heart.

4. Types of Beta Blockers: There are different types of beta blockers, including non-selective and selective beta blockers:

   - Non-selective beta blockers: These block both beta-1 and beta-2 receptors. Examples include propranolol and nadolol. They are often used for conditions such as angina, migraines, or essential tremors.

   - Selective beta blockers: These primarily block beta-1 receptors and have fewer effects on beta-2 receptors. Examples include atenolol, metoprolol, and bisoprolol. They are commonly used in patients with hypertension or certain heart conditions.

5. Additional Benefits: Beta blockers have additional benefits beyond blood pressure control. They are often prescribed for patients with certain heart conditions, such as heart failure, as they can improve symptoms, reduce hospitalizations, and prolong survival. Beta blockers may also help prevent recurrent heart attacks and manage symptoms in patients with angina.

6. Combination Therapy: Beta blockers can be used alone or in combination with other antihypertensive medications to achieve better blood pressure control. They are often combined with other classes of medications such as diuretics, ACE inhibitors, or ARBs.

7. Side Effects: Beta blockers are generally well-tolerated, but they can cause side effects in some individuals. Common side effects may include fatigue, dizziness, slowed heart rate, cold hands and feet, and sexual dysfunction. They may also mask the symptoms of low blood sugar in diabetic patients.

8. Precautions: Beta blockers should be used with caution in patients with certain medical conditions, such as asthma, chronic obstructive pulmonary disease (COPD), or heart block. They may interact with other medications, so it's important to inform your healthcare provider about all the medications you are taking.

It's important to take beta blockers exactly as prescribed by your healthcare provider. Regular follow-up visits are essential to monitor blood pressure, heart rate, and any potential side effects. Your healthcare provider will determine the most appropriate medication, dose, and treatment plan based on your individual needs, medical history, and response to treatment.

B. Combination therapy

Combination therapy for hypertensive patients involves the use of two or more antihypertensive medications from different classes to achieve better blood pressure control. It is a common approach when single-agent therapy does not adequately lower blood pressure or when the patient has specific indications for multiple medications. Here are some key points about combination therapy for hypertensive patients:

1. Improved Blood Pressure Control: Combining different classes of antihypertensive medications can enhance the effectiveness of treatment by targeting multiple mechanisms that contribute to high blood pressure. Each medication acts through a different pathway, allowing for a synergistic effect in lowering blood pressure.

2. Multiple Targets: Hypertension is a complex condition influenced by various factors, including blood volume, vascular resistance, hormone levels, and kidney function. Different classes of antihypertensive medications target these different factors, allowing for a comprehensive approach to blood pressure management.

3. Individualized Treatment: Combination therapy allows healthcare providers to tailor the treatment to the individual needs of the patient. Medications from different classes can be selected based on the patient's comorbidities, risk factors, and response to treatment.

4. Classes of Medications: The choice of medications for combination therapy depends on various factors, including the patient's medical history, concurrent medical conditions, and potential drug interactions. Common classes of antihypertensive medications used in combination therapy include diuretics, ACE inhibitors, ARBs, beta blockers, calcium channel blockers, and others.

5. Fixed-Dose Combination Products: Some antihypertensive medications are available as fixed-dose combination products, which combine two or more drugs into a single pill. These products simplify the medication regimen, improve adherence, and provide the convenience of taking multiple medications at once.

6. Side Effects and Adverse Reactions: Combination therapy may increase the risk of side effects and adverse reactions compared to monotherapy. It is important for healthcare providers to monitor patients closely for any adverse effects, including interactions between medications and any potential exacerbation of side effects.

7. Individual Response and Titration: Each patient may respond differently to combination therapy. The dosages of individual medications may need to be adjusted, and additional medications may be added or removed based on the patient's response and blood pressure goals.

8. Regular Monitoring: Regular follow-up visits are crucial to monitor blood pressure, assess the effectiveness of the combination therapy, and adjust the treatment plan as needed. Blood tests, such as renal function and electrolyte levels, may also be monitored to ensure the medications are well-tolerated.

Combination therapy should be prescribed and monitored by a healthcare provider experienced in managing hypertension. The specific combination of medications will depend on individual patient factors and may evolve over time as treatment progresses. It is important for patients to adhere to their prescribed regimen, attend regular follow-up appointments, and communicate any concerns or side effects to their healthcare provider.

1. Two-drug combinations

There are several two-drug combinations commonly used for the treatment of hypertension. These combinations typically involve medications from different classes to target multiple mechanisms involved in blood pressure regulation. Here are some examples of two-drug combinations for hypertensive patients:

1. ACE Inhibitor or ARB + Diuretic: Combining an ACE inhibitor or an angiotensin receptor blocker (ARB) with a diuretic is a common and effective combination. ACE inhibitors and ARBs help relax blood vessels, while diuretics promote the excretion of excess fluid and salt from the body. Examples of this combination include lisinopril/hydrochlorothiazide and losartan/hydrochlorothiazide.

2. ACE Inhibitor or ARB + Calcium Channel Blocker (CCB): This combination is often used when blood pressure is not adequately controlled with an ACE inhibitor or ARB alone. CCBs help relax and widen blood vessels, complementing the effects of ACE inhibitors or ARBs. Examples include amlodipine/valsartan and enalapril/amlodipine.

3. Diuretic + CCB: Combining a diuretic with a calcium channel blocker can be effective in lowering blood pressure. Diuretics promote fluid and salt excretion, while CCBs relax blood vessels. This combination is often used when a patient requires additional blood pressure reduction. Examples include hydrochlorothiazide/amlodipine and chlorthalidone/amlodipine.

4. Diuretic + Beta Blocker: Combining a diuretic with a beta blocker can be useful in patients with certain conditions, such as heart failure or angina. Diuretics reduce fluid volume, and beta blockers lower heart rate and contractility. This combination helps reduce the workload on the heart and lower blood pressure. Examples include hydrochlorothiazide/propranolol and chlorthalidone/metoprolol.

5. Beta Blocker + CCB: Combining a beta blocker with a calcium channel blocker is often used when blood pressure is not adequately controlled with a single medication. Beta blockers reduce heart rate and contractility, while CCBs relax blood vessels. This combination is particularly beneficial for patients with conditions such as angina or certain arrhythmias. Examples include atenolol/amlodipine and metoprolol/verapamil.

6. ACE Inhibitor + Beta Blocker: Combining an ACE inhibitor with a beta blocker can be beneficial for certain patients, particularly those with heart failure or a history of heart attack. ACE inhibitors help dilate blood vessels and reduce strain on the heart, while beta blockers lower heart rate and improve cardiac function. Examples include lisinopril/metoprolol and enalapril/carvedilol.

It's important to note that the specific combination therapy prescribed will depend on the individual patient's characteristics, comorbidities, and response to treatment. The choice of combination therapy should be made by a healthcare provider experienced in managing hypertension, considering factors such as efficacy, potential side effects, and drug interactions. Regular follow-up visits are essential to monitor blood pressure, adjust dosages, and assess the response to treatment.

2. Three-drug combinations

In certain cases, hypertensive patients may require three medications to achieve optimal blood pressure control. Three-drug combinations are often used when blood pressure is not adequately controlled with two medications or when the patient has significant hypertension and multiple risk factors. Here are some examples of three-drug combinations for hypertensive patients:

1. ACE Inhibitor or ARB + Diuretic + Calcium Channel Blocker (CCB): This combination is commonly prescribed when blood pressure remains high despite treatment with an ACE inhibitor or ARB plus a diuretic. Adding a calcium channel blocker helps to further lower blood pressure by relaxing blood vessels. Examples include lisinopril/hydrochlorothiazide/amlodipine and losartan/hydrochlorothiazide/amlodipine.

2. ACE Inhibitor or ARB + Diuretic + Beta Blocker: Combining an ACE inhibitor or ARB with a diuretic and a beta blocker is often used in patients with hypertension and other cardiovascular conditions such as heart failure or a history of heart attack. This combination targets multiple mechanisms involved in blood pressure regulation and cardiac function. Examples include

lisinopril/hydrochlorothiazide/metoprolol and losartan/hydrochlorothiazide/carvedilol.

3. Diuretic + Beta Blocker + Calcium Channel Blocker (CCB): This combination is commonly prescribed in hypertensive patients who require additional blood pressure reduction. The diuretic promotes fluid and salt excretion, the beta blocker lowers heart rate and contractility, and the calcium channel blocker relaxes blood vessels. Examples include hydrochlorothiazide/metoprolol/amlodipine and chlorthalidone/metoprolol/verapamil.

4. Diuretic + Calcium Channel Blocker (CCB) + Alpha Blocker: This combination is sometimes used when blood pressure is not sufficiently controlled with other two-drug combinations. The diuretic promotes diuresis, the calcium channel blocker relaxes blood vessels, and the alpha blocker reduces peripheral resistance by blocking alpha-adrenergic receptors. Examples include hydrochlorothiazide/amlodipine/doxazosin and chlorthalidone/amlodipine/prazosin.

5. ACE Inhibitor or ARB + Calcium Channel Blocker (CCB) + Alpha Blocker: This combination is used to address high blood pressure that is not adequately controlled with other two-drug combinations. The ACE inhibitor or ARB helps dilate blood vessels, the calcium channel blocker relaxes

blood vessels, and the alpha blocker reduces peripheral resistance. Examples include lisinopril/amlodipine/doxazosin and losartan/amlodipine/prazosin.

It's important to note that the specific combination therapy prescribed will depend on the individual patient's characteristics, comorbidities, and response to treatment. The choice of combination therapy should be made by a healthcare provider experienced in managing hypertension, considering factors such as efficacy, potential side effects, and drug interactions. Regular follow-up visits are essential to monitor blood pressure, adjust dosages, and assess the response to treatment.

C. Special considerations

Hypertensive patients may have specific considerations that need to be taken into account in their management. These considerations include the following:

1. Underlying Medical Conditions: Hypertensive patients often have other medical conditions, such as diabetes, kidney disease, or cardiovascular disease. These conditions may require additional medications or specific treatment approaches. Healthcare providers need to consider the overall health status of the patient and tailor the treatment plan accordingly.

2. Age: Older adults may require different treatment approaches due to age-related changes in the body and potential interactions with other medications they may be taking. Blood pressure targets may also differ based on age and the presence of other conditions, such as frailty or cognitive impairment.

3. Pregnancy: Hypertension during pregnancy requires special attention. Some antihypertensive medications are not recommended during pregnancy due to potential harm to the fetus. Pregnant women with hypertension need close monitoring and may require specific medications, such as

methyldopa or labetalol, which are considered safe in pregnancy.

4. Medication Interactions: Hypertensive patients often have other medications for concurrent conditions. Healthcare providers need to carefully consider potential interactions between antihypertensive medications and other drugs the patient is taking to avoid adverse effects or reduced effectiveness.

5. Side Effects and Tolerability: Some individuals may experience side effects from antihypertensive medications, such as dizziness, fatigue, or sexual dysfunction. It's important to monitor patients for these side effects and adjust the treatment plan as needed. In some cases, alternative medications or lower dosages may be necessary.

6. Lifestyle Factors: Hypertensive patients should be encouraged to adopt a healthy lifestyle, including regular physical activity, a balanced diet, weight management, smoking cessation, and stress reduction. Lifestyle modifications can have a significant impact on blood pressure control and overall cardiovascular health.

7. Ethnic and Racial Considerations: Certain ethnic and racial groups may have a higher prevalence of hypertension and different responses to specific antihypertensive medications.

Healthcare providers should be aware of these differences and consider them when selecting treatment options.

8. Patient Adherence: Adherence to the prescribed treatment plan is crucial for effective blood pressure control. Healthcare providers should assess patients' understanding of their medications, address any barriers to adherence, and provide support and education to promote compliance.

9. Regular Monitoring: Hypertensive patients require regular monitoring of blood pressure to assess the effectiveness of treatment and make any necessary adjustments. Additionally, monitoring other parameters such as renal function, electrolyte levels, and lipid profiles may be important for overall cardiovascular risk management.

Each hypertensive patient is unique, and their management should be individualized based on their specific needs and circumstances. It's important for patients to maintain regular follow-up visits with their healthcare provider to ensure ongoing monitoring, adjustment of treatment if necessary, and to address any concerns or questions.

1. Hypertension in pregnancy

Hypertension in pregnancy refers to high blood pressure that occurs during pregnancy. It is a significant medical condition that can have implications for both the mother and the baby. There are several types of hypertension that can occur during pregnancy:

1. Gestational Hypertension: This is a form of high blood pressure that develops after 20 weeks of pregnancy and resolves after delivery. It is characterized by elevated blood pressure without the presence of protein in the urine or other signs of organ damage.

2. Chronic Hypertension: Chronic hypertension is diagnosed when a woman has high blood pressure before pregnancy or before 20 weeks of gestation. It can persist after delivery and requires ongoing management.

3. Preeclampsia: Preeclampsia is a condition characterized by high blood pressure and signs of damage to other organ systems, typically the kidneys and liver. It can occur after 20 weeks of pregnancy and can be accompanied by proteinuria (protein in the urine). Preeclampsia can be severe and may progress to eclampsia, which involves seizures.

4. Eclampsia: Eclampsia is a severe and potentially life-threatening complication of preeclampsia. It is characterized by the onset of seizures or coma in a woman with preeclampsia.

Hypertension in pregnancy requires careful management to ensure the well-being of both the mother and the baby. Here are some key considerations:

1. Regular Blood Pressure Monitoring: Blood pressure should be monitored regularly throughout pregnancy to detect and manage hypertension. This can involve regular check-ups with healthcare providers or self-monitoring at home with a blood pressure cuff.

2. Medications: In some cases, medication may be necessary to control high blood pressure during pregnancy. Certain antihypertensive medications, such as methyldopa and labetalol, are considered safe for use during pregnancy. However, the choice of medication should be made by a healthcare provider, taking into consideration the specific needs of the mother and the potential effects on the baby.

3. Monitoring for Complications: Pregnant women with hypertension may be at increased risk for complications such as preeclampsia, growth restriction of the baby, placental

abruption, and preterm birth. Close monitoring of the mother and the baby is essential to detect and manage these complications early.

4. Lifestyle Modifications: Lifestyle modifications, including a healthy diet, regular physical activity, weight management, and stress reduction, can be beneficial in managing hypertension during pregnancy. It's important for pregnant women to follow the guidance of their healthcare provider regarding appropriate exercise and dietary recommendations.

5. Fetal Monitoring: Regular fetal monitoring, such as ultrasound examinations and non-stress tests, may be recommended to assess the well-being of the baby.

6. Delivery Planning: The timing and mode of delivery may need to be carefully considered in women with hypertension in pregnancy. In some cases, early delivery may be necessary to protect the health of the mother or the baby.

Hypertension in pregnancy requires close monitoring and management by healthcare professionals experienced in high-risk obstetrics. It's important for pregnant women with hypertension to maintain regular prenatal care visits, follow their healthcare provider's recommendations, and report any concerning symptoms promptly. With appropriate management, the risks associated with hypertension in pregnancy can be minimized, and the health outcomes for both the mother and the baby can be improved.

2. Hypertension in older adults

Hypertension, or high blood pressure, is a common health condition that affects many older adults. Managing hypertension in older adults requires special consideration due to the unique characteristics of this population. Here are some important points to understand about hypertension in older adults:

1. Prevalence: Hypertension becomes more common with advancing age. The age-related increase in blood pressure is attributed to various factors, including arterial stiffness, reduced elasticity of blood vessels, and changes in the renin-angiotensin-aldosterone system. As a result, a significant proportion of older adults are affected by hypertension.

2. Impact on Health: Hypertension in older adults is associated with an increased risk of cardiovascular diseases, including heart attacks, strokes, heart failure, and kidney disease. It can also contribute to cognitive decline and the development of other age-related health conditions. Therefore, effective management of hypertension is crucial to reduce the risk of these complications.

3. Blood Pressure Targets: Blood pressure targets for older adults may differ from those for younger individuals. The American Heart Association (AHA) and the American College of Cardiology (ACC) recommend a target blood pressure of less than 130/80 mmHg for most older adults without significant comorbidities. However, individualized treatment goals should be determined in consultation with a healthcare provider, taking into account the overall health status of the older adult, comorbidities, and functional status.

4. Comorbidities and Polypharmacy: Older adults often have multiple comorbidities, such as diabetes, kidney disease, and cardiovascular conditions. These comorbidities can influence the choice of antihypertensive medications and treatment strategies. Additionally, older adults are more likely to be taking multiple medications, which can increase the risk of drug interactions and adverse effects. Careful consideration of potential drug interactions and regular medication reviews are essential to ensure safe and effective management.

5. Medication Selection: The choice of antihypertensive medications in older adults should take into account factors such as efficacy, safety, tolerability, and the presence of specific comorbidities. Commonly prescribed medications include diuretics, calcium channel blockers, ACE inhibitors, and ARBs. However, individualized treatment plans should be

based on the specific needs and characteristics of the older adult.

6. Adverse Effects: Older adults may be more susceptible to the adverse effects of certain antihypertensive medications. For example, orthostatic hypotension (a sudden drop in blood pressure upon standing) can be more pronounced in older adults, particularly with medications such as alpha-blockers or certain diuretics. Close monitoring for side effects and regular follow-up visits are important to address any concerns and make necessary adjustments to the treatment plan.

7. Regular Monitoring: Regular blood pressure monitoring is essential in older adults with hypertension. It allows healthcare providers to assess the effectiveness of treatment, make necessary adjustments, and monitor for any complications or adverse effects. Home blood pressure monitoring can also be useful to track blood pressure trends and assist in treatment decisions.

8. Lifestyle Modifications: Lifestyle modifications play a crucial role in the management of hypertension in older adults. These include adopting a healthy diet (such as the DASH diet), regular physical activity, weight management, sodium restriction, limiting alcohol consumption, and stress reduction. Encouraging and supporting older adults in making

sustainable lifestyle changes can contribute to improved blood pressure control.

9. Comprehensive Geriatric Assessment: Older adults with hypertension may benefit from a comprehensive geriatric assessment, especially if they have multiple comorbidities or functional impairments. This assessment evaluates various domains of health, including physical, cognitive, and functional status, to develop a holistic treatment plan that addresses the unique needs of the individual.

3. Hypertension in patients with comorbidities (e.g., diabetes, renal disease)

Hypertension often coexists with other chronic conditions such as diabetes and renal disease. Managing hypertension in patients with comorbidities requires a comprehensive and tailored approach to address the specific needs and challenges associated with these conditions. Here are some considerations for managing hypertension in patients with comorbidities:

1. Individualized Treatment Goals: The treatment goals for blood pressure control in patients with comorbidities may differ from those without additional conditions. Guidelines, such as those from the American Diabetes Association or the National Kidney Foundation, provide specific recommendations for blood pressure targets in patients with diabetes or renal disease. Individualized treatment goals should be established in consultation with healthcare providers, considering the overall health status, age, and specific comorbidities of the patient.

2. Medication Selection: The choice of antihypertensive medications should consider the presence of comorbidities. Certain medications may have additional benefits beyond

blood pressure control that can be advantageous for patients with specific conditions. For example:

- Diabetes: Medications such as ACE inhibitors, ARBs, and certain calcium channel blockers (dihydropyridine type) have shown benefits in preserving kidney function and reducing the risk of cardiovascular events in patients with diabetes.

- Renal Disease: ACE inhibitors and ARBs are commonly used in patients with renal disease to protect kidney function and reduce proteinuria. However, their use should be carefully monitored for potential effects on renal function and electrolyte levels.

The choice of medication should be made based on the patient's specific needs, comorbidities, potential interactions, and the available evidence-based guidelines.

3. Close Monitoring: Patients with comorbidities require regular monitoring to assess the effectiveness of treatment and identify any potential complications. Monitoring may include blood pressure measurements, laboratory tests to evaluate kidney function and electrolyte levels, and assessments of disease-specific parameters (e.g., HbA1c levels in diabetes). Regular follow-up visits with healthcare providers are essential to monitor and adjust treatment plans as needed.

4. Lifestyle Modifications: Lifestyle modifications play a crucial role in managing hypertension and its associated comorbidities. Encouraging patients to adopt a healthy lifestyle, including a balanced diet, regular physical activity, weight management, and smoking cessation, can have positive effects on blood pressure control and overall health outcomes. In patients with diabetes, dietary modifications may also involve glycemic control through carbohydrate counting or specific dietary approaches recommended for diabetes management.

5. Collaborative Care: Managing hypertension and comorbidities often requires a multidisciplinary approach involving healthcare providers from different specialties. Collaborative care teams, including primary care physicians, endocrinologists, nephrologists, and other specialists, can work together to optimize treatment plans, address potential drug interactions, and manage complications related to the comorbid conditions.

6. Patient Education and Self-Management: Empowering patients to actively participate in their care is crucial. Providing education about hypertension, its relationship to comorbidities, and the importance of adherence to medication and lifestyle modifications can help patients take control of their health. Patient self-management strategies, such as self-monitoring of blood pressure or blood glucose levels (in

diabetes), can enhance patients' ability to manage their conditions effectively.

Managing hypertension in patients with comorbidities requires a holistic and patient-centered approach. It's important for healthcare providers to consider the specific needs of each patient, adhere to evidence-based guidelines, and promote shared decision-making to optimize blood pressure control and overall health outcomes. Regular communication, monitoring, and adjustments to the treatment plan are essential to ensure the best possible management of both hypertension and the associated comorbidities.

Chapter 4

IV. Monitoring and Follow-up

Monitoring and follow-up are crucial aspects of managing hypertension to ensure optimal blood pressure control and to detect any potential complications or treatment adjustments needed. Here are key points regarding the monitoring and follow-up of hypertension:

1. Blood Pressure Measurement: Regular blood pressure measurements are the cornerstone of hypertension monitoring. It's important to use accurate and validated blood pressure measurement devices. Blood pressure should be measured in a quiet, comfortable environment, with the patient in a relaxed state and after at least 5 minutes of rest. Multiple measurements at different visits are typically needed to establish an accurate blood pressure reading.

2. Blood Pressure Targets: Blood pressure targets are determined based on various factors, including age, presence of comorbidities, and individual patient characteristics. The target blood pressure level is usually set in consultation with healthcare providers, adhering to guidelines from professional organizations, such as the American Heart Association (AHA) or the European Society of Cardiology (ESC).

3. Frequency of Follow-up Visits: The frequency of follow-up visits depends on the severity of hypertension, the stability of blood pressure control, and the presence of any associated comorbidities. Generally, patients with well-controlled blood pressure may require follow-up visits every 3 to 6 months, while those with more complex or uncontrolled hypertension may need more frequent visits.

4. Medication Adjustments: Follow-up visits allow healthcare providers to assess the effectiveness of the current treatment plan and make necessary adjustments. Medication dosages may need to be modified, or additional medications may be added to achieve blood pressure goals. Close monitoring of blood pressure and any associated side effects is essential during these adjustments.

5. Lifestyle Modification Guidance: Follow-up visits provide an opportunity for healthcare providers to discuss and reinforce lifestyle modifications, such as adopting a healthy diet, engaging in regular physical activity, weight management, sodium restriction, reducing alcohol consumption, and smoking cessation. Patient education and ongoing support are important to promote sustained lifestyle changes.

6. Assessment of Treatment Adherence: Follow-up visits are an opportunity to assess patient adherence to the prescribed treatment regimen. Healthcare providers can inquire about any challenges or barriers to adherence and provide counseling or support to improve treatment compliance.

7. Monitoring of Comorbidities: Patients with hypertension often have other comorbidities, such as diabetes, renal disease, or cardiovascular conditions. Follow-up visits allow for the monitoring of these conditions, including appropriate laboratory tests, assessments of disease-specific parameters (e.g., glycemic control in diabetes), and the adjustment of treatment plans as needed.

8. Communication and Patient Engagement: Open and effective communication between healthcare providers and patients is crucial during follow-up visits. Healthcare providers should encourage patients to actively participate in their care, address any concerns or questions, and provide education and support to enhance patient engagement in their hypertension management.

9. Home Blood Pressure Monitoring: In certain cases, healthcare providers may recommend home blood pressure monitoring as an adjunct to office measurements. Home monitoring provides additional data and can help detect white coat hypertension (elevated blood pressure in medical

settings) or masked hypertension (normal office blood pressure, but elevated at home). It can also promote patient engagement and self-management.

Regular monitoring and follow-up visits allow healthcare providers to assess the effectiveness of treatment, make necessary adjustments, provide ongoing education and support, and detect any complications or emerging issues. It is essential for patients to adhere to scheduled follow-up visits and maintain open communication with their healthcare providers to optimize blood pressure control and overall cardiovascular health.

A. Blood pressure goals

Blood pressure goals refer to the target blood pressure levels that healthcare providers aim to achieve in the management of hypertension. These goals are typically based on guidelines provided by professional organizations, such as the American Heart Association (AHA), the European Society of Cardiology (ESC), or the National Institute for Health and Care Excellence (NICE). However, it's important to note that blood pressure goals may vary depending on individual patient factors, comorbidities, and treatment response. Here are general blood pressure goals for hypertension management:

1. Normal Blood Pressure: The goal for blood pressure is to achieve normal levels whenever possible. Normal blood pressure is typically defined as less than 120/80 mmHg.

2. Elevated Blood Pressure: For individuals with elevated blood pressure, which is systolic blood pressure (the top number) between 120-129 mmHg and diastolic blood pressure (the bottom number) less than 80 mmHg, lifestyle modifications are recommended to prevent progression to hypertension.

3. Stage 1 Hypertension: The target blood pressure for most individuals with stage 1 hypertension (systolic blood pressure of 130-139 mmHg or diastolic blood pressure of 80-89 mmHg) is generally set at less than 130/80 mmHg.

4. Stage 2 Hypertension: For patients with more severe hypertension (stage 2 hypertension), characterized by systolic blood pressure of 140 mmHg or higher or diastolic blood pressure of 90 mmHg or higher, the target blood pressure is often set at less than 130/80 mmHg, but individualized goals may be considered based on patient characteristics.

5. Specific Populations and Comorbidities: Blood pressure targets may vary for certain populations or individuals with specific comorbidities. For example:

  - Older Adults: The AHA and the ESC recommend a blood pressure target of less than 130/80 mmHg for most older adults without significant comorbidities. However, individualized treatment goals should be determined based on the overall health status, comorbidities, and functional status of the older adult.

  - Diabetes: In patients with diabetes, the recommended blood pressure target is typically less than 130/80 mmHg. However, individualized goals may be considered based on the patient's age, presence of microvascular complications, and overall health status.

- Chronic Kidney Disease (CKD): For patients with CKD, the blood pressure target is generally less than 130/80 mmHg. However, individualized goals may be considered based on the severity of kidney disease and the presence of proteinuria.

It's important to consult with a healthcare provider to determine the appropriate blood pressure goal for each individual based on their specific circumstances.

It's essential to note that blood pressure goals should be approached on an individual basis, considering factors such as age, comorbidities, and treatment response. The ultimate aim is to achieve blood pressure levels that minimize the risk of cardiovascular events and associated complications while considering the patient's overall health and individualized treatment plan. Regular monitoring and follow-up visits with healthcare providers are important to assess treatment effectiveness, adjust medication regimens if necessary, and ensure blood pressure control within the target range.

B. Frequency of monitoring

The frequency of monitoring hypertension depends on several factors, including the severity of hypertension, the stability of blood pressure control, the presence of comorbidities, and the patient's overall health status. Here are some general guidelines for the frequency of monitoring:

1. New Diagnosis or Medication Initiation: When a patient is newly diagnosed with hypertension or when antihypertensive medication is initiated or adjusted, more frequent monitoring is typically necessary. This helps assess the response to treatment and determine the effectiveness of the medication. In such cases, blood pressure may be monitored at least every 2-4 weeks initially.

2. Stable Blood Pressure Control: Once blood pressure is well-controlled and stable, less frequent monitoring may be appropriate. For most patients with stable blood pressure control, follow-up visits every 3-6 months are common. However, individualized plans should be determined based on the patient's specific circumstances and the healthcare provider's judgment.

3. Uncontrolled Hypertension or Comorbidities: Patients with uncontrolled hypertension or those with comorbidities that

require tight blood pressure control may require more frequent monitoring. This allows healthcare providers to assess the effectiveness of the current treatment plan, make necessary adjustments, and address any emerging issues promptly.

4. Age and Comorbidity Considerations: Older adults and patients with additional comorbidities, such as diabetes, kidney disease, or cardiovascular conditions, may require more frequent monitoring due to their increased cardiovascular risk. The presence of these comorbidities often necessitates closer monitoring and adjustment of treatment plans as needed.

5. Home Blood Pressure Monitoring: In certain cases, healthcare providers may recommend home blood pressure monitoring as an adjunct to office measurements. Home monitoring can provide additional data and help assess blood pressure patterns over time. This can be particularly useful for individuals with white coat hypertension (elevated blood pressure in medical settings) or masked hypertension (normal office blood pressure but elevated at home). Home blood pressure monitoring may require more frequent readings initially to establish accurate measurements and trends.

6. Individualized Assessment: The frequency of monitoring should be tailored to the specific needs of each patient. Healthcare providers should consider factors such as the

patient's response to treatment, the presence of target organ damage, the stability of blood pressure control, and any changes in health status. Individualized assessments should guide the decision-making regarding the appropriate frequency of monitoring.

It's important for patients to adhere to scheduled follow-up visits and maintain open communication with their healthcare providers. Regular monitoring of blood pressure allows for the assessment of treatment effectiveness, adjustment of medications if needed, evaluation of lifestyle modifications, and detection of any emerging issues or complications.

C. Lifestyle and medication adherence

Lifestyle and medication adherence are essential components of effective hypertension management. Here are some key points to note regarding lifestyle and medication adherence for hypertension patients:

1. Lifestyle Modifications:
   - Healthy Diet: Encourage patients to adopt a healthy eating plan, such as the DASH (Dietary Approaches to Stop Hypertension) diet, which emphasizes fruits, vegetables, whole grains, lean proteins, and low-fat dairy products. Limiting sodium (salt) intake and avoiding excessive saturated and trans fats is important.
   - Regular Physical Activity: Promote regular exercise and physical activity tailored to the patient's abilities and preferences. Aim for at least 150 minutes of moderate-intensity aerobic activity or 75 minutes of vigorous-intensity activity per week.
   - Weight Management: Advise patients to achieve and maintain a healthy weight through a combination of balanced eating, portion control, and regular physical activity.
   - Sodium Restriction: Encourage patients to reduce their sodium intake by avoiding processed and packaged foods,

reading food labels, and cooking meals at home using fresh ingredients.

- Limit Alcohol Consumption: Advise patients to consume alcohol in moderation, if at all. Men should limit their intake to two standard drinks per day, and women to one standard drink per day.

- Smoking Cessation: Provide resources and support to help patients quit smoking, as smoking can worsen hypertension and increase the risk of cardiovascular disease.

2. Medication Adherence:

- Education and Counseling: Provide patients with clear and understandable information about their medications, including their purpose, dosage, and potential side effects. Address any concerns or misconceptions they may have.

- Simplify Regimen: If possible, simplify the medication regimen by prescribing once-daily dosing or using fixed-dose combination products. This can help improve adherence by reducing the complexity of the medication routine.

- Regular Medication Schedule: Encourage patients to take their medications at the same time each day to establish a routine and reduce the likelihood of missed doses.

- Reminder Systems: Recommend the use of reminders, such as pill organizers, alarms, or smartphone applications, to help patients remember to take their medications as prescribed.

- Support Systems: Involve family members or caregivers in the medication adherence process, if appropriate, to provide support and reinforcement.

- Follow-up and Monitoring: Regularly assess medication adherence during follow-up visits. Ask patients about any difficulties they may be experiencing and address any barriers to adherence. Assess blood pressure control to determine the effectiveness of the medication regimen.

3. Patient Engagement:

- Shared Decision-Making: Involve patients in the treatment decision-making process, discussing the benefits and potential side effects of medications and lifestyle modifications. Encourage patients to take an active role in their care and express any concerns or preferences they may have.

- Addressing Barriers: Identify and address barriers to adherence, such as cost, medication side effects, forgetfulness, or difficulty understanding instructions. Work collaboratively with patients to find solutions to these challenges.

- Regular Communication: Maintain open lines of communication with patients, providing ongoing support, answering questions, and addressing any issues that may arise. Encourage patients to contact healthcare providers with any concerns or difficulties they encounter.

Lifestyle modifications and medication adherence are crucial for effective blood pressure control and reducing the risk of complications associated with hypertension. By focusing on patient education, support, and engagement, healthcare providers can help patients make sustainable lifestyle changes and adhere to their medication regimens, leading to improved outcomes and better overall cardiovascular health.

Chapter 5

V. Resistant Hypertension

Resistant hypertension is a term used to describe high blood pressure that remains above target levels despite the use of multiple antihypertensive medications. It is estimated that around 10-20% of patients with hypertension have resistant hypertension. Resistant hypertension is an important condition to identify and manage appropriately, as it can be associated with a higher risk of cardiovascular events and complications. Here are some key points regarding resistant hypertension:

1. Definition: Resistant hypertension is generally defined as the failure to achieve blood pressure control (usually defined as a target of less than 130/80 mmHg) despite the use of optimal doses of three or more antihypertensive medications, including a diuretic.

2. Potential Causes and Contributing Factors:
   - Inadequate medication regimen: Non-adherence to medications, improper dosing, or ineffective combinations of

antihypertensive medications can contribute to poor blood pressure control.

- Secondary causes: Resistant hypertension can be caused by underlying medical conditions, such as kidney disease, hormonal disorders (e.g., primary aldosteronism), obstructive sleep apnea, or renal artery stenosis. Identifying and treating these underlying conditions is crucial.

- Lifestyle factors: Unhealthy lifestyle choices, including poor diet, excessive sodium intake, sedentary behavior, obesity, and excessive alcohol consumption, can make blood pressure control more challenging.

- Medication-related factors: Certain medications, such as nonsteroidal anti-inflammatory drugs (NSAIDs), oral contraceptives, or corticosteroids, can interfere with blood pressure control and contribute to resistant hypertension.

- White coat hypertension or masked hypertension: Resistant hypertension may be due to misclassification of blood pressure readings in medical settings (white coat hypertension) or underestimation of blood pressure at clinic visits (masked hypertension). Ambulatory blood pressure monitoring can help identify these conditions.

3. Evaluation and Management:

- Thorough assessment: It is crucial to conduct a comprehensive evaluation to identify possible causes and contributing factors for resistant hypertension. This may include a review of the patient's medication regimen, assessment of lifestyle factors, screening for secondary causes, and ambulatory blood pressure monitoring to confirm the diagnosis.

- Medication optimization: Review the medication regimen to ensure optimal doses, proper combinations, and adherence to the prescribed medications. Consider adjustments in medication dosages, adding or switching medications, or using combination therapy to achieve better blood pressure control.

- Lifestyle modifications: Emphasize the importance of lifestyle modifications, including a healthy diet, regular physical activity, weight management, sodium restriction, alcohol moderation, and smoking cessation. These lifestyle changes can have a significant impact on blood pressure control, particularly in resistant hypertension.

- Addressing underlying causes: If an underlying cause or secondary hypertension is identified, appropriate treatment or referral to a specialist may be necessary to address the specific condition.

- Collaboration and specialist input: In challenging cases of resistant hypertension, consultation with a hypertension specialist, nephrologist, or endocrinologist may be beneficial to optimize management and address specific underlying causes.

- Patient engagement and education: Provide ongoing support, education, and encouragement to patients with resistant hypertension. Help them understand the importance of adherence to medications and lifestyle modifications to achieve better blood pressure control and reduce the risk of cardiovascular complications.

Managing resistant hypertension requires a comprehensive and individualized approach, taking into account potential contributing factors and addressing underlying causes. Regular follow-up visits, close monitoring, and collaboration among healthcare providers are crucial to optimize treatment strategies and improve blood pressure control in patients with resistant hypertension.

A. Definition and prevalence

A. Definition and prevalence of hypertension:

1. Definition: Hypertension, also known as high blood pressure, is a chronic medical condition characterized by elevated blood pressure in the arteries. Blood pressure is measured using two numbers: systolic pressure (the top number) and diastolic pressure (the bottom number). Hypertension is typically defined as having a systolic blood pressure of 130 mmHg or higher and/or a diastolic blood pressure of 80 mmHg or higher.

2. Prevalence: Hypertension is a common health condition worldwide and a major public health concern. According to the World Health Organization (WHO), in 2019, approximately 1.13 billion people had hypertension globally. The prevalence varies across countries and populations. Factors such as age, ethnicity, lifestyle habits, and socioeconomic status can influence the prevalence of hypertension.

   - Age: Hypertension becomes more prevalent with advancing age. As individuals age, the risk of developing hypertension increases.

- Ethnicity: Certain ethnic groups have a higher prevalence of hypertension. For example, African Americans tend to have higher rates of hypertension compared to other racial/ethnic groups.

- Lifestyle Factors: Unhealthy lifestyle habits, such as a poor diet (high in sodium and low in fruits and vegetables), physical inactivity, excessive alcohol consumption, and smoking, can contribute to the development and prevalence of hypertension.

- Socioeconomic Factors: Socioeconomic factors, including income level, education, and access to healthcare, can also influence the prevalence of hypertension. Disparities in hypertension prevalence exist among different socioeconomic groups.

It is important to note that hypertension is often referred to as a "silent killer" because it usually does not cause noticeable symptoms. However, if left uncontrolled, hypertension can lead to serious health complications, including heart disease, stroke, kidney disease, and other cardiovascular conditions. Regular blood pressure monitoring, lifestyle modifications, and appropriate medical treatment are crucial in the management and prevention of hypertension-related complications.

B. Evaluation and workup

The evaluation and workup of hypertension involve a comprehensive assessment to determine the underlying causes, evaluate organ damage, assess cardiovascular risk, and develop an appropriate treatment plan. Here are key components of the evaluation and workup of hypertension:

1. Medical History: A detailed medical history is obtained, including information about symptoms, family history of hypertension or cardiovascular disease, past medical conditions, medications, and lifestyle habits.

2. Blood Pressure Measurement: Accurate measurement of blood pressure is essential. Multiple measurements should be taken on different occasions to confirm the diagnosis and establish baseline blood pressure levels.

3. Physical Examination: A thorough physical examination is conducted to assess for signs of target organ damage and identify any secondary causes of hypertension. This may include examining the heart, lungs, abdomen, and assessing for evidence of end-organ damage.

4. Laboratory Tests:

- Basic Metabolic Panel: This includes tests to evaluate kidney function, electrolyte levels (such as sodium and potassium), and glucose levels.

- Lipid Profile: Assessing lipid levels (such as cholesterol and triglycerides) helps determine the overall cardiovascular risk.

- Urinalysis: A urinalysis may be performed to detect proteinuria, which can indicate kidney damage.

- Hemoglobin A1c: This test is performed to assess long-term blood sugar control in individuals with diabetes or suspected diabetes.

- Thyroid Function Tests: Thyroid disorders can contribute to hypertension, so thyroid function tests may be ordered if indicated.

- Additional Tests: Depending on the clinical presentation, other tests such as renal function tests, aldosterone/renin ratio, or sleep studies for sleep apnea may be considered.

5. Ambulatory Blood Pressure Monitoring (ABPM): ABPM involves wearing a portable blood pressure monitor that takes multiple blood pressure readings over a 24-hour period. ABPM helps evaluate blood pressure variability, detect white coat hypertension (elevated blood pressure in medical settings), and assess nocturnal blood pressure patterns.

6. Echocardiogram: In certain cases, an echocardiogram may be performed to assess the structure and function of the heart and detect any signs of hypertensive heart disease.

7. Additional Evaluation for Secondary Hypertension:
   - Renal Imaging: Imaging studies such as ultrasound, CT scan, or MRI may be performed to evaluate the kidneys for conditions like renal artery stenosis.
   - Endocrine Workup: If secondary hypertension is suspected, specialized testing may be conducted to evaluate hormonal abnormalities (e.g., aldosterone, cortisol levels) or conditions such as pheochromocytoma or Cushing's syndrome.
   - Sleep Studies: Sleep studies (polysomnography) may be recommended to assess for obstructive sleep apnea, which can contribute to hypertension.

8. Cardiovascular Risk Assessment: Evaluating cardiovascular risk involves assessing additional risk factors such as smoking, obesity, diabetes, lipid levels, age, and family history. Calculating risk scores, such as the Framingham Risk Score or ASCVD (atherosclerotic cardiovascular disease) risk calculator, helps determine the individual's risk of developing cardiovascular complications.

The evaluation and workup of hypertension aim to identify any underlying causes, assess target organ damage, evaluate cardiovascular risk, and guide treatment decisions. The findings from these evaluations help healthcare providers develop an individualized treatment plan, including lifestyle modifications, medication choices, and ongoing monitoring of blood pressure and associated conditions.

C. Management strategies

The management of hypertension involves a comprehensive approach that includes lifestyle modifications and, if necessary, pharmacological interventions. The primary goals of hypertension management are to lower blood pressure to target levels, reduce cardiovascular risk, and prevent or manage complications. Here are key management strategies for hypertension:

1. Lifestyle Modifications:
   - Healthy Diet: Encourage patients to adopt a healthy eating plan, such as the DASH (Dietary Approaches to Stop Hypertension) diet, which emphasizes fruits, vegetables, whole grains, lean proteins, and low-fat dairy products. Limiting sodium (salt) intake and avoiding excessive saturated and trans fats is important.
   - Regular Physical Activity: Promote regular exercise and physical activity tailored to the patient's abilities and preferences. Aim for at least 150 minutes of moderate-intensity aerobic activity or 75 minutes of vigorous-intensity activity per week.
   - Weight Management: Advise patients to achieve and maintain a healthy weight through a combination of balanced eating, portion control, and regular physical activity.

- Sodium Restriction: Encourage patients to reduce their sodium intake by avoiding processed and packaged foods, reading food labels, and cooking meals at home using fresh ingredients.

- Limit Alcohol Consumption: Advise patients to consume alcohol in moderation, if at all. Men should limit their intake to two standard drinks per day, and women to one standard drink per day.

- Smoking Cessation: Provide resources and support to help patients quit smoking, as smoking can worsen hypertension and increase the risk of cardiovascular disease.

2. Pharmacological Treatment:

- Antihypertensive Medications: Depending on the patient's blood pressure levels, overall health, and presence of comorbidities, healthcare providers may prescribe antihypertensive medications to lower blood pressure. Commonly prescribed medications include diuretics, beta-blockers, ACE inhibitors, ARBs, calcium channel blockers, and others. The choice of medication depends on individual patient factors and may require a trial-and-error process to find the most effective and well-tolerated treatment.

- Medication Adherence: Emphasize the importance of medication adherence to ensure consistent blood pressure control. Educate patients about their medications, including dosage, potential side effects, and the importance of taking them as prescribed. Address any concerns or barriers to adherence and provide support to enhance medication compliance.

3. Regular Monitoring and Follow-up:
   - Blood Pressure Monitoring: Regular monitoring of blood pressure is essential to assess the effectiveness of the treatment plan and make necessary adjustments. Encourage patients to monitor their blood pressure at home using a validated device and maintain a record to share with healthcare providers during follow-up visits.
   - Follow-up Visits: Schedule regular follow-up visits to evaluate blood pressure control, assess medication adherence, address any concerns or side effects, and provide ongoing support and education. The frequency of follow-up visits depends on the patient's blood pressure control, comorbidities, and individual needs.

4. Individualized Treatment Approach:
   - Consider Comorbidities: Take into account any comorbidities, such as diabetes, kidney disease, or cardiovascular conditions, when managing hypertension. Optimize treatment strategies to address these conditions and reduce overall cardiovascular risk.
   - Personalized Treatment Goals: Individualize blood pressure targets based on patient characteristics, overall health, and presence of comorbidities. Determine appropriate

treatment goals in consultation with the patient and consider evidence-based guidelines.

5. Lifestyle and Risk Factor Management:
   - Ongoing Education and Support: Continually educate and support patients in maintaining healthy lifestyle modifications, medication adherence, and other risk factor management strategies.
   - Multidisciplinary Care: Collaborate with other healthcare professionals, such as dietitians, nurses, or pharmacists, to provide comprehensive care and support patients in achieving

Chapter 6

VI. Hypertensive Emergencies

Hypertensive emergencies, also known as hypertensive crises, are situations in which severely elevated blood pressure (usually systolic blood pressure above 180 mmHg and/or diastolic blood pressure above 120 mmHg) is associated with acute end-organ damage. These emergencies require immediate medical attention to prevent or manage potentially life-threatening complications. Here are key points regarding hypertensive emergencies:

1. Types of Hypertensive Emergencies: Hypertensive emergencies are classified into two types based on the presence or absence of acute end-organ damage:
   - Hypertensive Urgency: In hypertensive urgency, there is severe elevation of blood pressure without acute target organ damage. Although blood pressure is significantly elevated, there is no immediate threat to organ function.
   - Hypertensive Emergency: In hypertensive emergency, there is severe elevation of blood pressure along with evidence of acute target organ damage. This can involve organs such as the brain (hypertensive encephalopathy), heart (acute myocardial infarction, heart failure), kidneys (acute kidney injury), eyes (retinopathy), or other organs.

2. Symptoms and Signs: Hypertensive emergencies may present with various symptoms depending on the organ(s) affected. These can include severe headache, visual changes, chest pain, shortness of breath, confusion, neurological deficits, seizures, severe anxiety, and signs of heart failure or kidney dysfunction.

3. Immediate Management:
  - Hospitalization: Hypertensive emergencies generally require hospital admission for close monitoring and immediate management.
  - Rapid Blood Pressure Reduction: In the setting of a hypertensive emergency, it is essential to lower blood pressure promptly but cautiously to prevent further end-organ damage. Intravenous antihypertensive medications are typically used to achieve controlled blood pressure reduction over a period of hours.
  - Individualized Treatment: The choice of antihypertensive medications and the rate of blood pressure reduction depend on several factors, including the severity of end-organ damage, the presence of comorbidities, and the patient's overall clinical condition. Medications commonly used in hypertensive emergencies include intravenous vasodilators (e.g., nitroglycerin, sodium nitroprusside), calcium channel blockers (e.g., nicardipine, clevidipine), or beta-blockers (e.g., labetalol).

- Monitoring and Supportive Care: Close monitoring of vital signs, organ function, and urine output is crucial. Additional supportive measures may be necessary, such as supplemental oxygen, cardiac monitoring, or dialysis in the case of acute kidney injury.

4. Underlying Causes and Evaluation:

- Identifying the underlying cause of the hypertensive emergency is important to guide appropriate management. Common causes include medication non-compliance, kidney disease, pheochromocytoma, acute adrenal insufficiency, or eclampsia in pregnant women.

- Evaluation typically involves laboratory tests (e.g., renal function, electrolytes, cardiac enzymes), electrocardiogram (ECG), chest X-ray, and possibly imaging studies (e.g., brain CT scan, echocardiogram) to assess organ damage and determine the underlying cause.

5. Long-term Management:

- After stabilization of the hypertensive emergency, a comprehensive evaluation and management plan for chronic hypertension should be established. This includes lifestyle modifications, initiation or adjustment of antihypertensive medications, and regular follow-up to ensure blood pressure control and prevent future hypertensive crises.

- Patient education regarding medication adherence, lifestyle modifications, and the importance of regular follow-up is crucial to prevent recurrence of hypertensive emergencies.

Hypertensive emergencies are serious medical conditions that require immediate attention. Timely recognition, appropriate management, and identifying and treating the underlying cause are vital

A. Definition and clinical features

Hypertensive emergencies refer to situations in which severely elevated blood pressure is accompanied by acute end-organ damage. These emergencies are characterized by severely elevated systolic blood pressure (typically above 180 mmHg) and/or diastolic blood pressure (typically above 120 mmHg). Hypertensive emergencies require immediate medical attention to prevent or manage potentially life-threatening complications.

Clinical features of hypertensive emergencies can vary depending on the organs involved and the extent of end-organ damage. The symptoms and signs may include:

1. Headache: Severe and persistent headache is a common symptom of hypertensive emergencies, particularly in cases of hypertensive encephalopathy (brain involvement).

2. Visual Changes: Vision disturbances, such as blurred vision or visual loss, may occur due to retinopathy or optic nerve involvement.

3. Chest Pain: Chest pain can occur in cases of acute myocardial infarction (heart attack) or acute coronary syndrome associated with severely elevated blood pressure.

4. Shortness of Breath: Breathlessness or difficulty breathing may be present due to acute pulmonary edema (fluid accumulation in the lungs) secondary to severe hypertension.

5. Neurological Symptoms: Neurological deficits can range from mild confusion and dizziness to more severe symptoms such as seizures, focal neurological deficits (e.g., weakness or numbness in one side of the body), or altered mental status. These symptoms may indicate hypertensive encephalopathy or stroke.

6. Signs of Heart Failure: Hypertensive emergencies can lead to acute heart failure, resulting in symptoms such as rapid or irregular heartbeat, edema (swelling) in the legs or other parts of the body, and shortness of breath.

7. Signs of Kidney Dysfunction: Acute kidney injury (kidney dysfunction) may present with decreased urine output, swelling in the legs, and changes in laboratory tests indicating impaired kidney function.

It is important to note that hypertensive emergencies can have serious consequences if not promptly managed. Immediate medical attention is required to assess the severity of the condition, initiate appropriate treatment to lower blood pressure, and prevent further end-organ damage. Early recognition and timely intervention are crucial in improving patient outcomes and preventing complications associated with hypertensive emergencies.

B. Immediate management and treatment

Immediate management and treatment of hypertensive emergencies aim to rapidly and safely lower blood pressure while preventing or minimizing end-organ damage. The specific approach may vary depending on the severity of the emergency, presence of complications, and individual patient factors. Here are key components of immediate management and treatment:

1. Hospitalization and Monitoring:
   - Hospital Admission: Hypertensive emergencies generally require hospitalization for close monitoring, evaluation, and management.
   - Vital Signs Monitoring: Continuous monitoring of blood pressure, heart rate, oxygen saturation, and other vital signs is crucial to assess response to treatment and detect any changes or complications.
   - Electrocardiogram (ECG): An ECG helps evaluate cardiac function, detect any myocardial ischemia or arrhythmias, and guide treatment decisions.

2. Blood Pressure Reduction:
   - Gradual Reduction: Blood pressure should be lowered gradually over a period of hours to prevent rapid decreases that may compromise organ perfusion.

- Medications: Intravenous antihypertensive medications are typically used to achieve controlled blood pressure reduction. The choice of medication depends on the individual patient's clinical presentation, underlying cause, and specific considerations. Commonly used medications include:

- Intravenous Vasodilators: Nitroglycerin, sodium nitroprusside, or nicardipine can be administered to relax blood vessels and lower blood pressure.

- Beta-Blockers: Medications such as labetalol or esmolol may be used to reduce heart rate and blood pressure.

- Individualized Approach: The specific medications and dosages are tailored to the patient's condition and closely monitored to achieve appropriate blood pressure control while avoiding complications.

3. Evaluation and Treatment of Underlying Causes:

- Identification: Determining and addressing the underlying cause of the hypertensive emergency is essential for optimal management. Possible causes may include medication non-compliance, renal disease, pheochromocytoma, acute adrenal insufficiency, or eclampsia in pregnant women.

- Diagnostic Tests: Additional diagnostic tests, such as renal function tests, urine analysis, imaging studies (e.g., brain CT scan, echocardiogram), or hormonal assays, may be performed to assess organ damage, identify the underlying cause, and guide treatment decisions.

4. Supportive Care:

- Symptom Management: Treatment of specific symptoms or complications associated with hypertensive emergencies is important. For example, oxygen therapy may be administered for respiratory distress or intravenous diuretics for acute pulmonary edema.

- Organ Function Monitoring: Continuous monitoring of organ function, including cardiac and renal function, is necessary to detect any deterioration or changes that require intervention.

- Fluid Management: Fluid balance and electrolyte levels are carefully monitored and managed to maintain appropriate hydration and optimize organ function.

- Prevention of Complications: Aggressive blood pressure control and comprehensive management aim to prevent or minimize complications associated with hypertensive emergencies.

It is important to involve a multidisciplinary team, including physicians, nurses, and specialists, to provide comprehensive and coordinated care for patients with hypertensive emergencies. The management approach should be tailored to each individual's condition and guided by ongoing assessment, monitoring, and treatment adjustments to ensure optimal blood pressure control and prevent further end-organ damage.

Chapter 7

VII. Lifestyle and Alternative Therapies

In addition to medical treatment, lifestyle modifications and alternative therapies can play a significant role in managing hypertension. These approaches can help lower blood pressure, reduce cardiovascular risk, and complement conventional treatment. It's important to note that lifestyle modifications and alternative therapies should be used as adjuncts to medical management and under the guidance of a healthcare professional. Here are some lifestyle modifications and alternative therapies that can be beneficial for hypertensive patients:

1. Dietary Approaches:
   - DASH Diet: Encourage patients to follow the Dietary Approaches to Stop Hypertension (DASH) eating plan, which emphasizes fruits, vegetables, whole grains, lean proteins, and low-fat dairy products. This diet is rich in nutrients such as potassium, magnesium, and calcium, which can help lower blood pressure.
   - Sodium Restriction: Advise patients to limit their sodium (salt) intake to no more than 2,300 milligrams (mg) per day or even lower, depending on individual needs. This involves

avoiding processed and packaged foods, reading food labels for sodium content, and cooking meals at home using fresh ingredients.

- Potassium-Rich Foods: Encourage the consumption of potassium-rich foods, such as bananas, oranges, spinach, tomatoes, potatoes, and legumes. Potassium helps counteract the effects of sodium on blood pressure.

2. Weight Management:

- Achieve and Maintain a Healthy Weight: Emphasize the importance of weight management for individuals who are overweight or obese. Even a modest weight loss can have a significant impact on blood pressure reduction. Encourage a balanced diet, portion control, and regular physical activity to achieve and maintain a healthy weight.

3. Regular Physical Activity:

- Aerobic Exercise: Encourage patients to engage in regular aerobic exercise, such as brisk walking, cycling, swimming, or jogging. Aim for at least 150 minutes of moderate-intensity aerobic activity or 75 minutes of vigorous-intensity activity per week.

- Resistance Training: Incorporating resistance training, such as weightlifting or bodyweight exercises, can also be beneficial for blood pressure control and overall cardiovascular health.

- Consultation with Healthcare Provider: Prior to starting or intensifying an exercise program, it's important for hypertensive patients to consult with their healthcare provider to ensure that the chosen activities are safe and suitable for their individual circumstances.

4. Stress Management:

- Stress Reduction Techniques: Encourage patients to practice stress reduction techniques, such as deep breathing exercises, meditation, yoga, or mindfulness. These techniques can help lower blood pressure and promote overall well-being.

- Engaging in Relaxing Activities: Encourage patients to participate in activities they enjoy, such as hobbies, listening to music, spending time in nature, or engaging in creative pursuits, to help reduce stress levels.

5. Limit Alcohol Consumption:

- Moderate Alcohol Intake: Advise patients to limit alcohol consumption to moderate levels. This means no more than two standard drinks per day for men and one standard drink per day for women. Excessive alcohol intake can raise blood pressure and negate the potential benefits of other lifestyle modifications.

6. Quit Smoking:

- Smoking Cessation Support: Encourage and support hypertensive patients who smoke to quit smoking. Smoking damages blood vessels, raises blood pressure, and significantly increases the risk of cardiovascular diseases. Referral to smoking cessation programs or healthcare professionals specialized in smoking cessation can be beneficial.

7. Alternative Therapies:

- Relaxation Techniques: Practices like acupuncture, biofeedback, or relaxation exercises may help some individuals manage their blood pressure and reduce stress.

- Herbal Supplements: Certain herbal supplements, such as garlic extract, hawthorn extract, or omega-3 fatty acids, have been suggested to have potential blood pressure-lowering effects. However, it's important to note that these

A. Stress management and relaxation techniques

Stress management and relaxation techniques can be valuable strategies for hypertensive patients to reduce stress levels and potentially lower blood pressure. Chronic stress is known to contribute to elevated blood pressure and increased cardiovascular risk. By incorporating stress management and relaxation techniques into their daily routine, hypertensive patients can promote overall well-being and potentially improve blood pressure control. Here are some stress management and relaxation techniques that can be beneficial:

1. Deep Breathing Exercises:
   - Diaphragmatic Breathing: Encourage patients to practice deep breathing exercises, also known as diaphragmatic or belly breathing. This involves inhaling deeply through the nose, allowing the belly to rise, and exhaling slowly through the mouth. Deep breathing promotes relaxation and helps reduce stress.

2. Meditation and Mindfulness:
   - Mindfulness Meditation: Teach patients mindfulness meditation techniques, which involve focusing their attention on the present moment without judgment. This practice can help reduce stress, improve emotional well-being, and promote relaxation.

- Guided Imagery: Guided imagery involves visualizing peaceful and calming scenes to induce a state of relaxation and reduce stress.

3. Progressive Muscle Relaxation:
   - Progressive muscle relaxation involves systematically tensing and relaxing different muscle groups in the body. This technique helps release muscle tension, promote relaxation, and reduce stress.

4. Yoga and Tai Chi:
   - Yoga and tai chi are mind-body practices that combine physical postures, controlled breathing, and mental focus. These practices have been shown to reduce blood pressure, improve cardiovascular health, and promote overall well-being.

5. Exercise and Physical Activity:
   - Regular aerobic exercise, such as brisk walking, jogging, swimming, or cycling, can help reduce stress and lower blood pressure. Encourage patients to engage in physical activity they enjoy to help manage stress levels effectively.

6. Social Support and Connection:
   - Encourage patients to maintain social connections and seek support from family, friends, or support groups. Talking

and sharing experiences with others can help reduce stress and improve emotional well-being.

7. Time Management and Prioritization:
   - Assist patients in developing effective time management strategies and prioritizing tasks to reduce feelings of overwhelm and stress. This may involve setting realistic goals, delegating tasks when possible, and maintaining a healthy work-life balance.

8. Relaxation Techniques Throughout the Day:
   - Encourage patients to incorporate relaxation techniques into their daily routine. This can include taking short breaks for deep breathing exercises or mindfulness practice, engaging in hobbies or activities they enjoy, or finding moments of tranquility and calm throughout the day.

It's important to note that while these techniques can be beneficial, they are not meant to replace medical treatment or lifestyle modifications. Hypertensive patients should consult with their healthcare provider before incorporating new practices, especially if they have any underlying health conditions or concerns. Healthcare providers can provide guidance, support, and additional resources to help patients effectively manage stress and improve blood pressure control.

B. Dietary supplements and herbal remedies

Dietary supplements and herbal remedies are commonly used by individuals seeking alternative or complementary approaches to manage hypertension. However, it's important to note that the use of these products should be approached with caution and under the guidance of a healthcare professional. Here are some dietary supplements and herbal remedies that have been suggested to have potential effects on blood pressure:

1. Garlic:
   - Garlic supplements or raw garlic are believed to have potential blood pressure-lowering effects. Garlic may promote blood vessel dilation and have mild antihypertensive properties. However, the evidence is mixed, and more research is needed to establish its effectiveness in managing hypertension.

2. Hawthorn:
   - Hawthorn extract, derived from the hawthorn plant, has been used traditionally to support cardiovascular health. Some studies suggest that hawthorn extract may have modest antihypertensive effects. However, further research is needed to confirm its effectiveness and safety.

3. Omega-3 Fatty Acids:

   - Omega-3 fatty acids, commonly found in fish oil supplements, have been associated with cardiovascular benefits. They may help reduce blood pressure, improve lipid profiles, and have anti-inflammatory effects. However, the evidence regarding omega-3 supplementation for blood pressure reduction is not definitive, and the optimal dosage and formulation are still under investigation.

4. Coenzyme Q10 (CoQ10):

   - CoQ10 is an antioxidant naturally produced by the body, which plays a role in cellular energy production. Some studies suggest that CoQ10 supplementation may have a modest effect in reducing blood pressure, particularly in individuals with hypertension. However, more research is needed to establish its efficacy and optimal dosage.

5. Hibiscus:

   - Hibiscus tea or hibiscus extract has been associated with potential blood pressure-lowering effects. Some studies have shown that hibiscus may have a modest antihypertensive effect. However, more research is required to determine its efficacy and safety.

It's important to emphasize that while these dietary supplements and herbal remedies may have some potential benefits, they should not be considered as standalone treatments for hypertension. They should be used as adjuncts to lifestyle modifications and prescribed medications, and their use should be discussed with a healthcare professional. Some supplements may interact with medications or have side effects, and their quality and purity can vary among products.

It is recommended that individuals consult with a healthcare provider, such as a doctor, pharmacist, or registered dietitian, before starting any dietary supplement or herbal remedy, especially if they have pre-existing health conditions or are taking other medications. A healthcare professional can provide personalized guidance, evaluate potential risks and benefits, and ensure that these supplements are used safely and effectively in conjunction with conventional hypertension management strategies.

C. Complementary therapies (e.g., acupuncture)

Complementary therapies, such as acupuncture, are alternative treatment approaches that some individuals consider for managing hypertension. While research on the effectiveness of these therapies for hypertension is ongoing, it's important to note that they should be used as adjuncts to conventional medical treatment and under the guidance of a qualified healthcare professional. Here is information on acupuncture as a complementary therapy for hypertension:

Acupuncture:
1. Definition: Acupuncture is a traditional Chinese medicine practice that involves the insertion of thin needles into specific points on the body. It is believed to balance the flow of energy, known as Qi, along pathways called meridians.

2. Potential Benefits: Some studies suggest that acupuncture may have potential benefits for blood pressure management. It is believed to stimulate the release of endorphins, which can help relax blood vessels and potentially lower blood pressure. Acupuncture may also help reduce stress and promote relaxation, which can indirectly contribute to blood pressure control.

3. Research Findings: The research on acupuncture for hypertension is mixed, and more high-quality studies are needed to establish its effectiveness. Some studies have shown modest blood pressure-lowering effects of acupuncture, while others have not found significant benefits. It's important to note that individual responses to acupuncture may vary.

4. Safety Considerations: Acupuncture is generally considered safe when performed by a qualified and trained practitioner. The needles used are typically sterile, disposable, and single-use to minimize the risk of infection. However, it's important to consult with a healthcare professional before undergoing acupuncture, especially if you have any underlying health conditions or are taking medications.

5. Integration with Conventional Treatment: Acupuncture should be used as a complementary therapy alongside conventional medical treatment for hypertension. It should not be used as a substitute for prescribed medications or lifestyle modifications. It's important to inform your healthcare provider if you are considering acupuncture or any other complementary therapy, as they can provide guidance and ensure coordinated care.

6. Choosing a Qualified Practitioner: When seeking acupuncture treatment, it's important to choose a licensed and experienced acupuncturist who adheres to proper hygiene

practices. Consult with your healthcare provider for recommendations or seek practitioners who are certified by recognized acupuncture associations or regulatory bodies.

It's important to emphasize that the decision to pursue acupuncture or any other complementary therapy for hypertension should be made in consultation with a healthcare professional. They can provide personalized advice, consider individual circumstances, and help ensure that these therapies are used safely and appropriately alongside conventional management strategies.

Chapter 8

VIII. Conclusion and Future Directions

Hypertension is a prevalent health condition that requires ongoing management to reduce the risk of cardiovascular complications. The management of hypertension involves a multifaceted approach that includes lifestyle modifications, pharmacological interventions, and regular monitoring. Lifestyle modifications, such as adopting a healthy diet, engaging in regular physical activity, maintaining a healthy weight, limiting alcohol consumption, quitting smoking, and managing stress, play a crucial role in blood pressure control and overall cardiovascular health.

Pharmacological treatments, including various classes of antihypertensive medications, are prescribed based on individual patient characteristics and blood pressure levels. The selection of medications may involve single-drug therapy or combination therapy, depending on the patient's needs. Regular monitoring of blood pressure, evaluation of target organ damage, and assessment of cardiovascular risk are essential for optimizing treatment outcomes and preventing complications.

While lifestyle modifications and pharmacological interventions form the cornerstone of hypertension management, complementary therapies and alternative approaches, such as acupuncture and certain dietary supplements, may be considered as adjuncts. However, their use should be discussed with healthcare professionals and incorporated in a coordinated manner with conventional treatment.

Future directions in hypertension management include ongoing research to better understand the underlying mechanisms of hypertension, identify novel therapeutic targets, and refine treatment approaches. Additionally, personalized medicine and precision approaches, considering genetic, environmental, and individual factors, hold promise in tailoring treatment strategies to optimize blood pressure control and reduce cardiovascular risk.

Public health efforts should focus on raising awareness about hypertension, promoting healthy lifestyle habits, and enhancing access to healthcare services. Early detection, timely intervention, and effective management of hypertension can significantly reduce the burden of cardiovascular disease and improve overall health outcomes.

It is important for individuals with hypertension to actively engage in their own care, work closely with healthcare professionals, adhere to treatment plans, and maintain regular follow-up visits to monitor blood pressure and manage the condition effectively. By implementing a comprehensive and individualized approach to hypertension management, the aim is to achieve optimal blood pressure control, reduce the risk of complications, and enhance overall quality of life.